HEALING

THROUGH THE

VAGUS

NERVE

Quarto.com

© 2024 Quarto Publishing Group USA Inc.
Text © 2024 Amanda Armstrong

First Published in 2024 by Fair Winds Press, an imprint of The Quarto Group,
100 Cummings Center, Suite 265-D, Beverly, MA 01915, USA.
T (978) 282-9590 F (978) 283-2742

Fair Winds Press titles are also available at discount for retail, wholesale,
promotional, and bulk purchase. For details, contact the Special Sales Manager
by email at specialsales@quarto.com or by mail at The Quarto Group, Attn:
Special Sales Manager, 100 Cummings Center, Suite 265-D, Beverly, MA
01915, USA.

28 27 26 25 24   1 2 3 4 5

ISBN: 978-0-7603-8506-7

Digital edition published in 2024
eISBN: 978-0-7603-8507-4

Library of Congress Cataloging-in-Publication Data available.

Design: Sylvia Sporto
Page Layout: Burge Agency
Illustration: Eleanor Hardiman

Printed in China

The information in this book is for educational purposes only. It is not intended
to replace the advice of a physician or medical practitioner. Please see your
health-care provider before beginning any new health program.

HEALING
THROUGH THE
VAGUS
NERVE

Improve Your Body's Response to
ANXIETY, DEPRESSION, STRESS, and
TRAUMA Through Nervous System Regulation

AMANDA ARMSTRONG, MA
Founder and CEO of Rise as We

Foreword by Dr. Monique Andrews

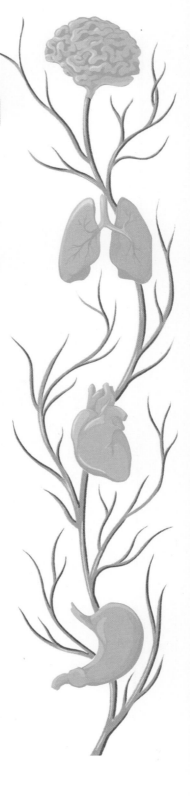

CONTENTS

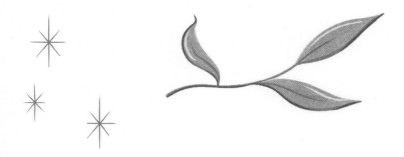

FOREWORD

Current statistics estimate that one-third of Americans will experience a period of anxiety or depression at least once in their lifetime. In a world where anxiety and depression are commonplace, so many are in search of a path to healing. *Healing Through the Vagus Nerve* is a guiding light on that journey, providing a holistic, trauma-informed approach to self-regulation that empowers those struggling with anxiety and depression.

As a long-time teacher and scholar of embodied neuroscience, I was delighted to find that very topic at the heart of this book's approach. It's a perspective that encourages us to explore our body as a vital component of our mental and emotional health. When we engage in exercises and practices that promote somatic awareness, we become more attuned to the sensations, tensions, and emotions within us. As we deepen this awareness, we enhance our ability to self-regulate our nervous system, reducing stress, anxiety, and other factors that contribute to the chaos of modern life.

The vagus nerve, sometimes called the *compassion nerve*, through its intricate network of connections, has the remarkable capacity to modulate our stress response and influence our emotional well-being. In *Healing Through the Vagus Nerve*, you'll discover how to activate and tone this crucial nerve, enabling it to effectively communicate with your body and brain, fostering a state of calm and equilibrium.

This book is not just for those facing health challenges but for anyone seeking a deeper connection with their body and emotions. It's for individuals who desire a toolset to enhance their overall well-being and to navigate the turbulent waters of life with grace and resilience. By engaging with the exercises and practices provided within these pages, you'll embark on a transformative journey that may not only heal your vagus nerve but also heal your soul.

While reading *Healing Through the Vagus Nerve*, you'll find yourself stepping onto a path that is not about a quick fix but about long-lasting transformation. This journey is an invitation to connect with your own inner wisdom and resilience, to unearth the latent potential within you. As you delve into these pages and immerse yourself in the practices, you will come to appreciate your body's innate wisdom and its capacity to heal and self-regulate.

The lessons and techniques you'll find—from yoga to breathwork to simple massage—are a testament to the remarkable potential for healing that resides within each one of us. Use them as an opportunity to learn how to foster self-awareness, embrace self-compassion, and engage in practices that can heal your vagus nerve. Through this journey, you may discover a profound sense of self and a life that is characterized by greater balance and emotional well-being.

May you approach this journey with an open heart, prepared to embrace the possibilities within. This book is an invitation to awaken your own inner healer. As you follow the path laid out within its pages, you may find not just relief from anxiety and depression but also a deep connection with your own healing potential.

With gratitude,
Dr. Monique Andrews | Embodied Neuroscientist
A Grateful Reader

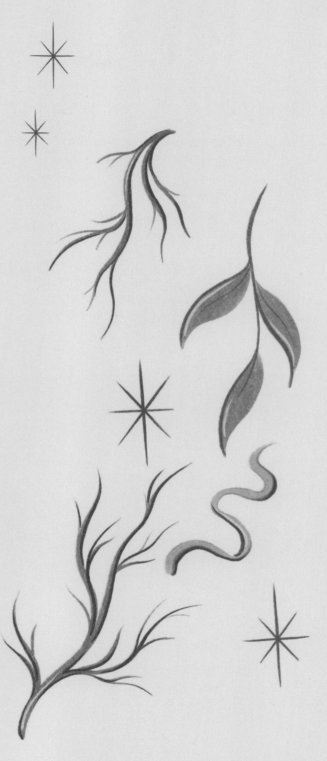

INTRODUCTION

I'll never forget the feeling I had the first time one of my clients said, "Oh my gosh, I'm not broken. This all makes perfect sense!" I've since seen this incredible "aha" moment hit for hundreds of clients and it never gets old. I find it fascinating that most often it comes not from years of therapy or big life changes but from simply beginning to understand how their nervous system works. Once the nervous system comes into focus, they realize their anxiety, their depression, and their symptoms are a natural result of their past lived experiences and current life stressors. This realization brings compassion and curiosity and paves the way for some of their deepest healing.

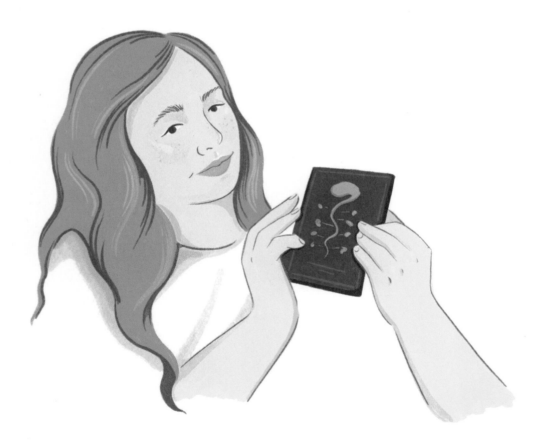

I believe that nervous system regulation is the foundation to all other healing, not just because I witness it every day with clients, but because of my own personal healing journey as well. There were many years I felt at war with my mind and body—and I didn't see a way out. When I finally got the courage to go to the doctor and ask for help, I wanted to better understand why I was struggling. Instead, like many of you have likely experienced, I left a few minutes later with a prescription. When I made my way to a therapist, it felt helpful to talk through things. However, I often left thinking, "Well, now what?" It felt frustrating to spend so much time talking about my struggles without having tangible tools to start feeling better.

I'm not bashing medication or therapy when I say that. There's a time and a place for most interventions. Different people need different things at different times, and I'm grateful for everything that supported me in my healing—medication and therapy both for a short time. But my reality was that those two mainstream options left gaping holes when it came to the support and healing that I wanted and needed. I remember the feeling of not knowing where else to turn.

Eventually, through countless hours of research, I found what I was missing: the connection between the mind and body. In the last decade of neuroscience and psychological research, we've learned that so much stress, trauma, anxiety, and depression actually lives in the body rather than in the brain. When it comes to the mind-body connection and nervous system regulation, the vagus nerve is key. It is the superhighway that supports mind-body communication, and 80 percent of those signals and information originate in the body. When the vagus nerve is optimal and functioning, overall mental and physical health improve in tangible and measurable ways. That means the nervous system, mainly the vagus nerve, is at the center of it all! As you begin to learn how this system functions, you can start working *with* it in a powerful and tangible way. The first part of this book focuses on building this understanding.

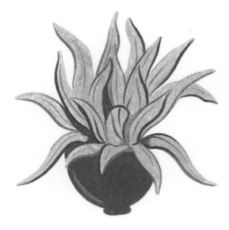

Training the Nervous System

Imagine you've just arrived at the gym. You walk in and see a 300-pound weight on the floor. Should you walk up to it, without training, and expect yourself to deadlift (or otherwise pick up) the 300-pound weight? Of course not! Most people wouldn't even try, and if you did, it makes sense that you might hurt yourself in that attempt. Yet so many people are doing the equivalent of trying to lift a 300-pound life of struggles and emotional distress with little to no training. No one taught you how to carry this load, so of course you're struggling! It feels hard and it's not your fault.

Just as you would train in the gym, there are powerful ways to train and leverage your physiology, your body, and your nervous system to influence and heal your psychology and your mind. There are ways to push back against your body's stress response in real time and increase your capacity to carry a heavier load. There are certain habits that hurt and others that heal. Knowing how your mind-body system works is the most powerful step in learning to work *with* it, and eventually train with it, instead of fighting against it.

This is a big part of the active work in this book, specifically the exercises in chapter 6. I'm confident that the education and tools I share on those pages will help you take steps to improve your mental and physical health through this sort of nervous system training—not just because they've worked for me, but because I've seen, and continue to see, them work for hundreds of clients in their journeys to reclaim their lives from anxiety and depression.

Personalize Your Plan

Training is all well and good, but again, just like at the gym, everyone starts at a different place and needs to keep their own limits and unique needs in mind when training. My goal for this book is not to simply share a list of "vagus nerve hacks," but to help you understand and build a relationship with *your* entire nervous system. Your vagus nerve plays a vital role in that system, but there is no "hacking" your way to healing. Instead, I'll lay a foundation of education that will empower you to personalize the tools and practices taught in this book.

Mental health looks different for everyone, and so will the solution. As I share what's worked for me and so many of my clients, I'll invite you to experiment and personalize it in a way that works for you. My clients each take their own approach to nervous system regulation through somatic practices, parts work, and personalized behavior change coaching that follows my four-phase neuroscience- and trauma-informed framework for healing (education, regulation, rewiring, and resourcing). I'll teach you more about this framework a little later in this book.

I can't provide a completely personalized approach through this book, of course. Still, I will try to support you in how to take what you're learning and create a practical application for your daily life. Read through these pages with personal interest. Take time to pause and ask, "How does what I just read apply to me? What does this look like in reflection to my life?" Personalization is going to be key to the impact you get from this book. My hope is that anyone can pick it up, better understand their vagus nerve and nervous system as a whole, and take tangible action to move toward healing.

How This Book Is Organized

I've organized the book in a way that takes you on a similar journey to the one I walk my clients through. In chapters 1 and 2, you'll learn more broadly about the role your nervous system and vagus nerve play in your mental and physical health. In chapters 3 and 4, I will guide you through how to personalize that new knowledge to help you better understand the current state of your unique nervous system and vagus nerve. Understanding the physiology and your current baseline is essential before you can jump into using any of the tools in a productive way. Then, in chapter 5, I give you a framework for how to regulate your nervous system and heal your vagus nerve in a personalized and strategic way. This is followed by chapter 6, which will provide a library of guided somatic and vagal toning exercises for you to come back to over and over again on your healing journey. Then, finally, in chapter 7, I provide some blueprints to get you started on creating your very own vagal toning routine to help you reconnect to your body, regulate your nervous system, and reclaim your life.

By the end of this book, I hope to give you not only hope and inspiration but also real-life tools and strategies. You'll learn the science that validates your struggle (and with each chapter, new pieces of this puzzle will fall into place). You will feel seen, heard, and supported, and you will come to realize that you are not broken. All of your symptoms (and maybe all of you!) make sense through this nervous system lens based on your past lived experiences, your current life circumstances, and the coping skills and resourcing you either have or lack.

I assure you, you can heal and you've come to the right place to learn how. This book will deconstruct what helps people heal through a nervous system, trauma-informed, mind-body lens and I will be with you every step of the way on your own personal journey.

Thanks for being here.

Amanda

WANT GUIDED SUPPORT WHILE READING THIS BOOK?

I created a video companion course with this in mind. In the course, I walk through each chapter of this book, providing additional context and questions to aid with reflection. It also includes videos to demonstrate many of the exercises in chapter 6. Just visit www.riseaswe.com/vagusnerve.

1

THE AUTONOMIC NERVOUS SYSTEM

The nervous system is the key to the body's incredible capacity to heal itself.

As the body's communication network, the nervous system plays a central role in every moment of our lives—from how we feel, think, and react to how well our body is physically functioning. Understanding how this system works and the role it plays in your well-being enables and empowers you to work *with* it to move toward healing instead of feeling like you're constantly fighting *against* your mind and body on that journey.

So often when people think about things like anxiety, depression, stress, or trauma, there is the tendency to say it may be "all in your head." However, the reality is that all of these things are rooted in the body. Thus, understanding, befriending, and regulating the nervous system can provide an alternative road map to healing.

Put another way: Have your health issues ever felt like a game of whack-a-mole? Just as you get a handle on one symptom, others seem to pop up in its place. That's probably because many modern medical practices focus on symptom management. We often find ourselves chasing from one symptom to the next with medication, operations, or other treatments. As helpful as all of these interventions may be, when you fail to zoom out and see how things are connected you may miss out on finding the common thread (and thus getting to the root cause).

The nervous system often lies at the heart of these various issues. Because the autonomic nervous system plays such a huge role in the body's important

functions—including circulation, digestion, immunity, respiration, and reproduction—when it is dysregulated, a lot can go wrong. Inversely, when you work to create a more regulated nervous system, largely through vagus nerve function, you can tap into your body's natural ability to heal. Many of your seemingly unrelated symptoms may begin to subside.

Here is a list of some common problems that can arise from or could be related to nervous system dysregulation: Chronic pain, jaw clenching, migraines, eye or facial tension, autoimmune conditions, anxiety, depression, PTSD, insomnia or other sleep disturbances, addiction, chronic exhaustion, chronic stress, dissociation, high blood pressure, poor digestion, IBS, constipation or diarrhea, low immunity, difficulty concentrating, poor memory, loss of interest in sex.

Have you experienced some of these symptoms? If so, read on because what follows in this book will be an invaluable guide to a new path toward long-term mental and physical health.

And while many of the chapters in this book provide a blueprint of how to work toward this goal, first I'd like to introduce you to, and help you understand, your nervous system in a functional way that has been helpful to so many of my clients. In this chapter, you'll find a quick anatomical and functional snapshot of how the autonomic nervous system functions. (I know some of this may seem nerdy, but you'll be grateful for this information later!)

THE AUTONOMIC NERVOUS SYSTEM

The nervous system is made up of the brain, brainstem, spinal cord, and nerves that branch off from the brain and spinal cord and extend to all parts of the body. Its number one job is to keep you alive. Your nervous system doesn't care whether you reach your goals or live a good life; every part of it is hardwired for the survival of your physical body. My focus in this book is on the autonomic nervous system. This is the part of our peripheral nervous system that handles involuntary bodily functions and gland regulation. It is responsible for the unconscious tasks important for survival, like heartbeat, blood pressure, breathing, digestion, and reproduction. The state of this system also significantly impacts mental health.

The autonomic nervous system has two systems that act somewhat like a seesaw of stress and de-stress. These two systems are parasympathetic and sympathetic. When the autonomic nervous system interprets our internal functioning and our external environment to be safe, it is in a parasympathetic, or relaxed, state. When it labels something as a problem or threat in any way, it activates a sympathetic state, also known as your body's stress response.

When the sympathetic state is activated, your body's physiology changes in a very real way. Your heart rate speeds up, blood gets pumped to your extremities, pupils enlarge, and muscles tense—your body mobilizes so that you can fight or flee from whatever the threat is. In this state, your body also turns down or off functions not needed for immediate survival: things like digestion, bladder control, reproduction, cognitive function, and various other things that can be returned to when things are safe and going well.

Ideally, you only shift into sympathetic activation temporarily and then quickly return to spend most your time in the parasympathetic state, feeling safe and connected—this is where our mind and body optimally function. Unfortunately, the fast-paced and stressful nature of modern-day society often creates the reverse reality, where you may be feeling stressed out far more often than relaxed. This is a major contributor to nervous system dysregulation.

Some primary causes of nervous system dysregulation are chronic stress, poor lifestyle habits, trauma, big life changes, environmental toxicity, and excessive inflammation. All of us experience ebb and flow through seasons of regulation and dysregulation; the key is in befriending the nervous system enough to work with it and see whether it is the common thread intertwining many of your seemingly unrelated symptoms.

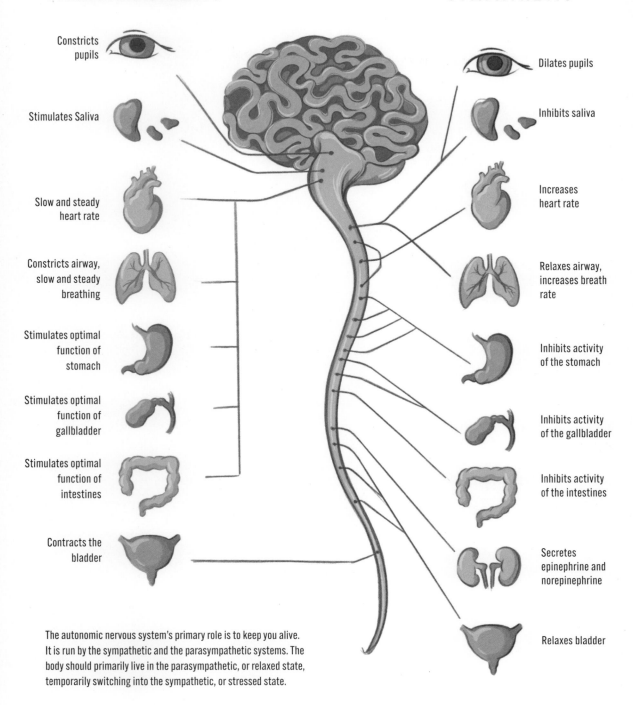

PARASYMPATHETIC

SYMPATHETIC

Constricts pupils

Dilates pupils

Stimulates Saliva

Inhibits saliva

Slow and steady heart rate

Increases heart rate

Constricts airway, slow and steady breathing

Relaxes airway, increases breath rate

Stimulates optimal function of stomach

Inhibits activity of the stomach

Stimulates optimal function of gallbladder

Inhibits activity of the gallbladder

Stimulates optimal function of intestines

Inhibits activity of the intestines

Contracts the bladder

Secretes epinephrine and norepinephrine

Relaxes bladder

The autonomic nervous system's primary role is to keep you alive. It is run by the sympathetic and the parasympathetic systems. The body should primarily live in the parasympathetic, or relaxed state, temporarily switching into the sympathetic, or stressed state.

The Sympathetic Nervous System

The sympathetic nervous system is most associated with the "fight-or-flight response." Its job is to activate and prepare your body to take action. This state isn't exclusively reserved for emergency situations, though. Your everyday life is a dance between parasympathetic and sympathetic. It's common for people to vilify this activated state because it is most associated with things like stress, danger, and anxiety, but it's equally involved in things like excitement, focus, and crushing a good workout. The problem is not activation: it's the amount of time you spend there. Many people wake up feeling stressed or anxious, having that seesaw already tilted toward the activation state, and then rarely, if ever, throughout the day feeling it tip back in the other direction to feeling calm and connected. If this is true for you, it's going to leave you exhausted and/or locked into being stressed out as your default state. The goal in nervous system regulation is to help you reset your default state to the parasympathetic state. This happens through understanding and working with this mind-body system to create more moments where you feel safe and capable, and to learn to recognize whether your stress responses appropriately reflect the situation at hand. If it doesn't, if you find yourself often overreacting or underreacting, then throughout this book I want to equip you with tools to change your response.

As humans, our stress response is immediate, coordinated, and generic. (Note: I will be using the terms *sympathetic activation* and *stress response* interchangeably.) To help you remember how quickly and automatically the sympathetic nervous system works, you can look to the root of the word *sympathetic*: it means "together or connection between parts." I find this an accurate description. The neurons that make up the sympathetic nervous system live in the thoracic and lumbar spinal cord (think *neck to navel*). As soon as stress of any kind is detected, within 500 milliseconds—half a second—the neurons in this system have deployed neurotransmitters, or chemical messengers, into the body to have your pupils dilate, inhibit digestion, increase heart rate and respiration, and more, as you can see in the graphic on page 15. The sympathetic nervous system stimulates functions needed for our fight-or-flight response and inhibits any functions not needed for survival. Later on, when I start talking about ways to manage stress, it's helpful to understand how quick and automatic this system is, because this means it's going to be very hard to *prevent* the stress response from happening. Thus, the best strategy often needs to be getting better at pushing back on it and intentionally turning on a relaxation response through the parasympathetic nervous system.

The Parasympathetic Nervous System

The parasympathetic nervous system is often referred to as the "rest and digest" or "social engagement" state. This state of safety and relaxation allows your body systems to reset and begin functioning optimally again. As I mentioned earlier, you want this as your default state, but my guess is that if you are picking up a book like this you may spend more time feeling stressed or anxious than rested and social.

This part of our nervous system originates in the brainstem and sacral spinal cord as well as in the pelvic area. The cranial nerves have direct lines to various features of your face, in particular your eyes.

Note: Starting on page 112, you'll learn some powerful tools to stretch and engage your eyes as a way to use certain entry points of the parasympathetic nervous system as levers that allow you to directly push back on the stress response in real time to help reset and feel more relaxed quite quickly.

Here's quick snapshot of the cranial nerves and their various functions.

The vagus nerve is the star of the show, as it makes up a huge part of the parasympathetic nervous system, innervating most major organs and playing a big role in mental health as well. Improving your understanding and function of the vagus nerve is one of the most powerful ways to combat stress and anxiety. Before we really get into the vagus nerve, though, I want to help you understand your nervous system as a whole in a more tangible and functional way (beyond the detailed scientific descriptions). As I do, I'll invite you to do some self-reflection to help you build awareness around *your* nervous system and the particular state it is in most often.

Nerve #	Name	Function
1st	Olfactory	Relays smell
2nd	Optic	Transmits visual information
3rd	Oculomotor	External muscles of the eye
4th	Trochlear	Also supplies muscles of the eyes
5th	Trigeminal	Chewing and sensation in the face
6th	Abducent	Controls lateral eye movement
7th	Facial	Muscles of facial expression, taste buds, sensations in fingers and toes, blinking
8th	Auditory	Hearing and balance
9th	Glossopharyngeal	Sensation, taste, and swallowing
10th	Vagus	The longest and most diverse cranial nerve with both sensory and motor responsibilities, innervating most major organs through the body
11th	Accessory	Supplies two neck muscles, sternomastoid and trapezius
12th	Hypoglossal	Muscles of the tongue and neck

A FUNCTIONAL UNDERSTANDING OF THE NERVOUS SYSTEM

Think of your nervous system like a computer that has a log of everything you've ever experienced from conception to today. Sure, it logs the good stuff, but the nervous system is hardwired for survival, so it puts a little red flag on all the files containing situations in your life where you felt unsafe, didn't get your needs met, experienced rejection or shame, and so on. It does this to make sure that if anything happens in your future that feels familiar to one of these past situations you will be more prepared.

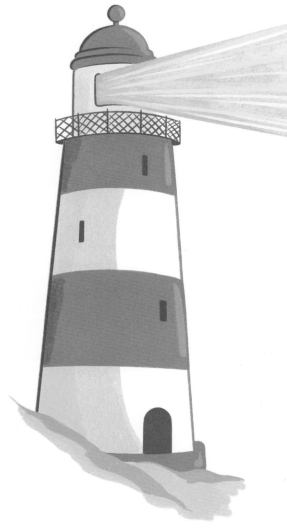

Now, in the present moment, your nervous system operates more like a lighthouse. Imagine that strong beam of light, constantly scanning the environment. Your nervous system, using something called *neuroception*, is constantly scanning situations in your life and checking back in with that database to see whether anything in your current situation or environment feels familiar to a time in your past when you didn't feel safe or get your needs met. Anytime something pings as familiar, your internal alarm system (aka *sympathetic state*) gets triggered.

Most of the situations I'm talking about are stored in something called your "implicit memory" (as opposed to "explicit memory"). Implicit memory, sometimes referred to as *unconscious memory*, is made up of the things people don't purposely try to remember and is often a body-based, somatic, or *feeling*-based memory. This is in contrast to explicit memories, which are conscious and can be verbally explained.

Much of what makes up how your nervous system perceives a situation in the present moment is based on things you experienced in your past that are now stored in your implicit memory, which relies less on the facts about a situation and more on how a situation makes you feel.

The key word with how the nervous system operates is in the word *feel*. You see, the nervous system speaks a somatic felt language, not a verbal one. Have you ever had a situation where you logically knew you were safe but you didn't *feel* safe? What's more, you still didn't feel any better no matter how many times you thought to yourself, "I'm fine, everything is fine, stop overreacting, I shouldn't feel this stressed or anxious ..." Again, this happens because your body doesn't speak a verbal language; it speaks a somatic language. Somatics is the language of *show me* I'm safe, don't *tell me* I'm safe. You will learn how to work in this language through various tools and practices shared in this book. It's the best way to communicate with your body when you want to turn on your relaxation response to show your nervous system you're safe. In fact, if you do this enough times, you can eventually rewire your nervous system to be less reactive and to reset after stressful situations more quickly.

This book will provide many different opportunities for you to not only get more acquainted with your nervous system but also to provide you conceptual and tangible ways to better navigate it. Navigating the nervous system means that you have the awareness to recognize what state you're in and an understanding of the tools that give you agency over that state. Agency to calm down when you've been activated, liven up when you're feeling tired or shut down, and how to source for the internal and external support needed. You'll learn the powerful ways in which your physiology drives your psychology, and also the tangible ways in which you can leverage your body systems, especially your vagus nerve, to powerfully heal as well. Understanding how to navigate your body states opens up your world, allowing you to be more fully present in situations and to feel more in control of how you show up.

As you'll soon learn, the activation (what we usually label "anxiety") or shut down (what is commonly labeled "depression") of your system is not any level of brokenness within you. What I hope you come to see is that oftentimes this activation or shutdown of your system may actually be a healthy response to an unhealthy circumstance—a healthy and protective response to what you've been through or are currently experiencing. As you learn to navigate the nervous system, or dare I say even befriend it, you can begin to see the positive intent behind your symptoms, states, and stories. Doing so opens up the doors to curiosity and self-compassion on your healing journey.

The more you understand how this mind-body system works, the more you can work *with* it toward healing. One of my favorite frameworks for functionally understanding the nervous system and how it impacts our daily life is through the polyvagal theory.

POLYVAGAL THEORY

In my practice, I turn often to Dr. Porges's polyvagal theory. Dr. Porges is a psychologist and behavioral neuroscientist who first introduced the polyvagal theory in 1994 as a link between the evolution of the autonomic nervous system and social behavior, and it emphasizes the importance of physiological state in the expression of behavior and psychology. The polyvagal theory introduces a three-part nervous system model and discusses how the vagus nerve directly impacts the communication and connection within the autonomic nervous system. I have found it to be an incredibly helpful framework for teaching clients to understand their anxiety and depression through a nervous system lens, and it gives them a tangible operating manual for their nervous system.

The three parts, or states, of the nervous system according to the polyvagal theory are:

- **Ventral Vagal:** This is a healthy parasympathetic state, also referred to as the "social engagement" state. When you are in this state, your nervous system is regulated and you feel calm, grounded, present, curious, and connected to yourself and others. As explained previously, this parasympathetic state is where all your bodily functions are operating optimally and you feel pretty good.

- **NOTE:** It's not important that you learn the official names of things in this book; it's just important that you understand the concepts enough to apply them to your daily life. So in the future I'll refer to this state in accessible terms like "regulation" or the "green zone."

- **Sympathetic:** This is a state of hyperarousal, or activation; it is your fight-or-flight response. Think about this like your nervous system's gas pedal; here your physiology is primed for mobilization. There's been a perceived stressor or threat and you need to accelerate into action to either fight off or flee from the stressor. Here, you'll feel worried, frustrated, angry, fearful, anxious, or panicked. In future discussion, I'll refer to this state as the "stress response," "activation," or "yellow zone."

- **Dorsal Vagal:** This is a state of hypoarousal, or shutdown; it is sometimes referred to as your freeze response, although there are others who consider the freeze response to be a state of extreme sympathetic activation plus dorsal vagal shutdown. Think about this like your nervous system pulling the emergency break when you need to immediately stop or shut down; here physiology is primed for immobilization. This happens when the nervous system has become so overwhelmed that it shuts down. You may feel flat, numb, helpless, dissociated, depressed, or hopeless. In future discussion, I'll refer to this state as "shutdown" or the "red zone."

The Autonomic Nervous System Ladder

Another leader in polyvagal theory and trauma, Deb Dana, encourages people to think about these states laid out on a ladder. Dorsal vagal is on the bottom, sympathetic activation is in the middle, and ventral vagal is at the top of the ladder. This ladder creates a predictable path that the nervous system moves through, in sequence. For example, you don't just jump from being at the top of the ladder in a regulated, ventral vagal state, to being at the bottom in a dorsal vagal, shutdown state. You must first pass through some mobilization in a sympathetic state, even if ever so briefly; this may go almost unnoticed. The same applies in reverse. If you find yourself in dorsal vagal shutdown, an immobilized state, before you can settle into the regulated state of ventral vagal you must first pass through some mobilization. I often work with clients who struggle with depression,

and after some time working together, they notice that their depression symptoms now feel more like anxiety. In our next session there's often a concern that something has gone wrong. This is when I'll refer them back to this ladder as a reminder that those shifts in symptoms from immobilization (depression) to mobilization (anxiety) often actually mean they're getting closer to a regulated state—that the work is having an effect, rather than anything going wrong. This is why understanding how your nervous system operates is so important to working with it in your healing journey. This autonomic nervous system ladder provides a map of sorts for how our nervous system states shift and how we move up and down this ladder, by activating either the sympathetic or the parasympathetic branch of the autonomic nervous system ladder in response to various stimuli throughout our day and life.

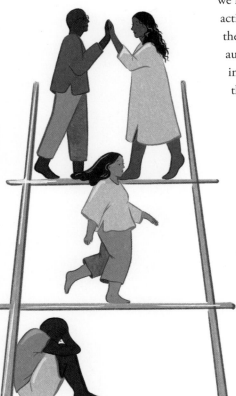

Ventral State:
Regulated, Safe
and Social

Sympathetic
State: Mobilized,
Flight or Flight

Dorsal State:
Immobilized,
Collapsed or
Shutdown

Zones of the Autonomic Nervous System

Another way of understanding how we move through the various nervous system states is to think about each state as a "zone," like I referenced in the descriptions of the polyvagal theory section. The green zone is where you are regulated, feeling safely connected to yourself and others; the yellow zone is a state of activation, where you are in your fight-or-flight survival response; and the red zone is a state of shutdown where you feel disconnected, depressed, or frozen.

To bring this to life even more, I often use something called the "stress bucket" to help clients understand the nervous system and how it responds to our thoughts and experiences, contributing to which zone, or nervous system state, you find yourself in at any given moment.

Imagine for a moment that you're standing at the top of a staircase holding a bucket. Now, you understand that you can only put so much in a bucket before it's either too heavy for you to carry or it starts to overflow. That bucket represents your nervous system's carrying capacity. When the stress load on your nervous system is light, your bucket is light. You're at the top of the staircase in that green zone feeling regulated, in control, and calm. As you, or life, add stressors, your bucket gets heavier and heavier, pushing you further and further down the staircase. Your first attempt to manage stress is usually your fight-or-flight response, in that yellow zone. But if the stressors are too big or last too long, you will get pushed even further down into your shutdown state.

The goal of nervous system regulation isn't to always stay in the green zone. Things happen in everyday life that move you through these various nervous system states. Instead, the goal of nervous system regulation is to have the tools to flexibly move up and down that staircase, between the different states. As you get better at noticing which state you are in, the more you can learn and apply specific tools to help you move your way back into the green zone, setting that as your baseline instead of feeling like you're stuck in a constant state of survival mode. Regulation happens by learning how to better manage the load in your bucket by either increasing your capacity to carry a heavier load or by decreasing the weight in the bucket. This happens through proactive and reactive nervous system regulation, much of which improves the overall function of the vagus nerve, which we will talk about later in this book.

To help you cultivate better interoception, or the ability to check in with yourself and know which state you're in based on body sensations, let's personalize what you've just learned.

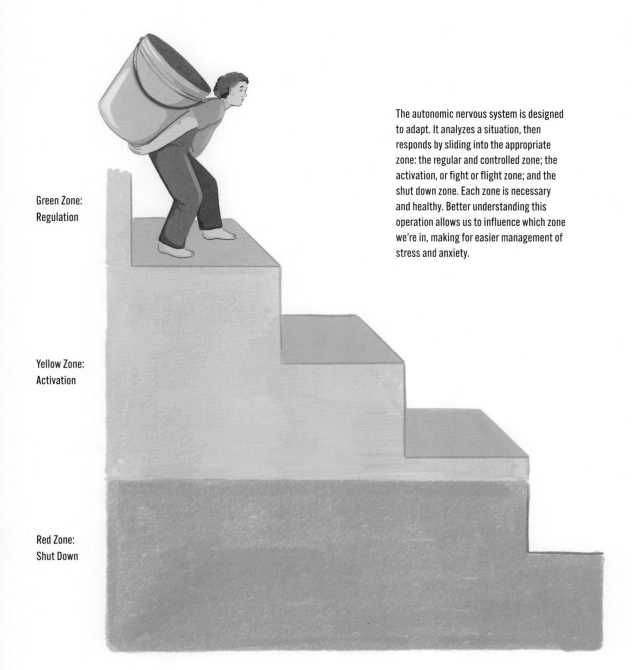

Green Zone:
Regulation

Yellow Zone:
Activation

Red Zone:
Shut Down

The autonomic nervous system is designed to adapt. It analyzes a situation, then responds by sliding into the appropriate zone: the regular and controlled zone; the activation, or fight or flight zone; and the shut down zone. Each zone is necessary and healthy. Better understanding this operation allows us to influence which zone we're in, making for easier management of stress and anxiety.

If you don't yet have the answers to those questions yet, that's okay. I'll support you in building more interoception throughout this book. One of the first things I invite clients to do, and I'd like to invite you now to try, is to swap out "anxiety" or "depression" with "activate" or "shut down" for the next month or so. For example, "I feel so anxious when I drive" becomes "I feel so activated when I drive" or "I hate feeling depressed" becomes "I hate feeling shut down." Doing this helps you tune in to your body-based experience of anxiety and depression, which increases your interoception and orients you to healing through this body-first approach. When it comes to regulating your nervous system, before you can jump into effectively changing anything, you first need to learn to speak the body's language, which happens through felt sensations rather than logical thinking. This reframe or relabeling is a really simple but impactful place to start to reorient you to this new lens of healing.

Again, the goal of regulating your nervous system isn't to live forever in the green zone. A regulated nervous system is a flexible nervous system, one that can move between states to meet the need of different situations or stressors while having the ability to return and reset to the green zone when that stressor has passed. You become dysregulated when there are too many stressors or you've spent so much time in either the red or yellow zone that it's become your default operating state because you didn't, and don't, have the tools to regulate and push back on your stress response in real time. I hope to help you change that by the end of this book.

HOW DYSREGULATION OCCURS

Nobody has the luxury of waiting until adulthood to learn how to get their needs met or stay safe in this world. That means much of the programming that runs the show in your life today was put together by a much younger version of you. Let's talk about how this happens.

A healthy stress cycle is when you get temporarily activated due to a specific stimuli or situation. Then, once that passes, you are able to discharge the no longer needed stress energy and reset into a state of regulation, feeling safe, calm, and capable. Children do not have the ability to self-regulate; in fact, most adults are still learning how to do this effectively. This means when a child is having a big emotion or experiencing a difficult situation, they are dependent on a calm and regulated adult to help their system settle and get that reset. When that isn't available, the nervous system often becomes overwhelmed. Instead of discharging that stress energy, it gets stored in the body. Layer by layer, each time your nervous system is overwhelmed, stress energy gets stored in the body, which creates a chronic state of nervous system dysregulation.

This can shrink something Dan Siegal, a clinical professor of psychiatry, calls the "window of tolerance." This simply refers to the zone in which you can function normally, where you handle stress well, and maintain an optimal level of arousal. When you are inside your window, you are able to learn, connect with others, make decisions, feel grounded, be curious, and think logically. Inside this window, you can feel a range of emotions and your nervous system remains regulated. (When I say "regulated" I mean that there's a natural tilting back and forth between that seesaw of stress and de-stress systems without ever feeling out of control or out of balance one way or the other.) This is synonymous with the "green zone" mentioned earlier.

However, if the stressors become too much, we get pushed outside our window in two ways:

- **Hyperarousal:** This is the fight-or-flight response, a sympathetic state, aka "yellow zone." Here you might have difficulty concentrating; be really reactive; and feel activated, angry, anxious, irritable, and panicky.

- **Hypoarousal:** This is an overactive parasympathetic state, aka "red zone." Here you might feel a sense of shutting down. You may feel flat or numb, dissociated, depressed, isolated, or helpless.

Individuals who have experienced chronic or traumatic stress tend to have a smaller window of tolerance, making it more difficult to regulate emotions and feel grounded. Understanding this concept helps explain why some people react more intensely to stress or certain situations than others. We all have different windows due to things like neurobiology, social support, environments, coping skills, stress, or trauma. And your window size can even vary from day to day. But the goal of most well-being work, and this book, is to help you increase the overall size of your window of tolerance. This should allow you to feel more in control of your mind, emotions, actions, and life.

Real-Life Example

A client of mine, we'll call her Michelle, couldn't understand why she was so anxious and reactive all the time. After working with me, she began to put pieces together that helped her make sense of it. Overall, she would describe her childhood as good and normal. Her parents didn't have the best relationship, but they were still together and she always had her basic needs met. She eventually reflected on the fact that as a child she was often sent to her room when she was upset, and she unconsciously understood being sent to her room to mean "I'm less lovable when I'm angry or upset." So, she learned to suppress these emotions, never allowing her to truly reset her nervous system in a healthy way, which trapped that stress energy in her body. Her dad also felt unpredictable, meaning sometimes something she did would make him mad and other times it wouldn't. She, again unconsciously, became hypervigilant, with her nervous system always staying on high alert to try to predict any subtle cues about the kind of mood her dad was in. Layer this in with some of her other experiences with school bullying, a car accident, and some other life events that wouldn't seem too out of the ordinary, and it all adds up. Without the balance of learning healthy ways of coping with or resolving these stressors, they contributed to patterns of chronic stress and nervous system dysregulation.

She eventually realized that she was still suppressing emotions. She felt uneasy while driving, second-guessed herself in relationships, and was often hyper-vigilantly surveying people and situations—assuming the worst or jumping to a worst-case scenario. Anytime something felt even vaguely familiar to her nervous system to how she felt in past overwhelming situations, she was immediately triggered and didn't have tools to navigate that. This kept a constant load on her nervous system, making her baseline nervous system state sympathetic activation, or the yellow zone. When this becomes a default state, feeling reactive or anxious can be a common baseline.

The point is that the current state of your nervous system is often a reflection of your past lived experience, combined with the stressors of your current life circumstances, offset by the coping skills or awareness you do or don't have to manage it all.

Children become adults who learn to self-regulate because it was modeled for them. Children become adults who are compassionate and kind to themselves in hard moments because adults were compassionate and kind to them in hard moments. Children become adults who can feel safe saying no, setting boundaries, and sharing their feelings when a loving parent shows them how to do these things. If you didn't have this as a child, it makes sense that you're struggling with it as an adult. The good news is that it's never too late to learn these things for yourself.

An Imbalance of Load & Capacity

Sometimes, like the example I just shared, dysregulation has roots in the past. Other times, dysregulation is a natural result of a stress bucket that's too full. A couple pages back, I mentioned that this "stress bucket" represents your nervous system's carrying capacity. What fills this bucket is anything and everything you navigate in your daily life: work stress, home responsibilities, relationships, hobbies, children, finances, decision making, lifestyle habits, thoughts, health, etc.

Does the load you're trying to manage outweigh your carrying capacity? Is that load pushing you down the nervous system ladder, down that staircase, or outside your window of tolerance? Sometimes you are simply carrying too much.

We often forget that our society has evolved much faster than our biology. Much of our biology is still primed for living life around a fire, eating berries, and sleeping in caves together. You weren't really ever meant to juggle all the things that modern life, or even your own expectations, demands of you.

In my coaching practice, we often help clients sort out whether their dysregulation or reaction to something is rooted in the past or if it was the last drop in their stress bucket. When your reaction seems disproportionate to the circumstance at hand, you can ask yourself: "Is this because I'm overwhelmed and my stress bucket is full? Or is it because I've been triggered based on a past experience?"

Are you feeling out of sorts after a call with your mom because it pinged an inner-child wound or because you're juggling a million things? Is your kids yelling and playing getting on your last nerve because you're underslept, undernourished, and overworked or because you weren't allowed to play and yell as a kid?

This may seem trivial, and some of you may be asking why it even matters. It matters because understanding the root of dysregulation helps set you on the more helpful path to regulation and healing.

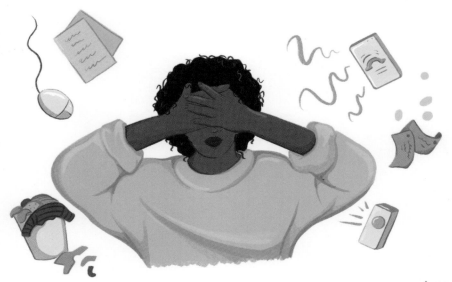

WHAT IS STRESS?

The one thing that keeps coming up in everything we've talked about so far is the stress response. Overall, the autonomic nervous system is the interplay, the seesaw, between the sympathetic and parasympathetic states via the turning on and off of our stress response.

These opposing systems for stress and de-stress are part of our hardwiring as humans.

In order to understand this dance between our sympathetic activation and parasympathetic relaxation responses, we need to understand stress. If ever there was a topic that brought together our mind-body relationship, it is stress.

Stress is nothing more than our body's natural and evolutionarily driven way of responding to a stressor. Okay, so what's a stressor? A stressor is anything that your brain or body decides requires attention or action. Two broad categories of stressors are:

- **Physical stressors:** These are stressors that put strain on the body in some way. Things like exercise, illness, noise, injury, environmental pollution, poor respiration, poor diet, chronic pain, very hot or cold temperatures, dehydration, natural disasters, and substance use are all examples.

- **Psychological stressors:** These are anything that we interpret as negative or threatening. Things like emotional stress (resentment, fear, grief, anger, loneliness), cognitive stress (information overload, worry, guilt, shame, self-criticism, finances, anxiety), perceptual stress (beliefs, worldview, roles, stories), relational difficulties, work stress, lack of social support, loss of employment, and lack of resources for adequate survival are all examples.

NOTE: Many people believe there is also a category of modern-day stressors that overlap categories, things like home life demands, traffic, social media, the news, prejudice, and social injustices.

As humans, we are great at facing challenges. We are hardwired for seeking out safety and solutions, but modern-day life has become so much more complex than our nervous systems were designed to handle.

Our stress response is generic, meaning that it wasn't designed for any one specific thing. It doesn't know that our society has evolved. It doesn't know, or care, whether stressors are outside us (like hearing sirens, getting a distressing text message, touching something hot, smelling smoke) or inside us (like remembering an argument you had with your mom, thinking about an upcoming test or presentation, viral infection, eating something spoiled). It responds all the same. Any input from inside or outside our body can be interpreted as a stressor, and the acute, short-term stress response is designed to combat all stressors in a similar way.

The stress response wasn't specifically designed for one thing or another, which enables it to quickly, and often, take over our entire mind-body system. But because it's generic in its response, it also gives us an advantage of controlling it once we better understand it. To do this, let's take a quick look at the difference between short-term and long-term stress.

Short-term, or acute, stress typically lasts anywhere from minutes to hours. This form of stress is an immediate response to a specific stressor. Once that has been handled, your adrenaline and cortisol levels diminish and your system returns to normal. And believe it or not, this kind of stress is actually good for us. Did you know that short-term stress actually primes your immune system to fight infection? When adrenaline is released, it signals parts of your immune system to release killer cells to combat bacterial and viral infections. Short-term stress also narrows your

focus, so it's not great at helping you make big picture decisions, but rather in accomplishing the specific task at hand. Normal amounts of the two primary stress hormones, adrenaline and cortisol, are necessary for survival. In fact, in many cases, the two hormones are beneficial to overall health and well-being. So where does it go awry? The problem is when stressor after stressor after stressor comes one after the other without you ever being able to fully reset: this is referred to as long-term stress.

Long-term, or chronic, stress is characterized by a consistent sense of feeling pressured or overwhelmed over a long period of time. No specific parameters have been put around chronic stress, but if you feel stressed more often than not, you likely fall into this category. This is the stress we most often hear about—and the one that medical research estimates is a cofactor in as much as 90 percent of illness and disease. We also know that chronic stress negatively impacts the functioning of the vagus nerve and is known to contribute to anxiety, depression, digestive problems, muscle tension, headaches, problems with memory and cognition, sleep problems, decreased immunity, high blood pressure, heart disease, and the list goes on and on. Chronic stress changes the shape and function of our brain and impacts almost every major function in our body. The good news is that we have the ability to mitigate these impacts when we better understand our stress response and nervous system as a whole, and your vagus nerve has a big role to play in that.

Managing stress, and dysregulation, is a matter of managing our capacity and load. If you're living life in a constant state of overwhelm and chronic stress, then something's got to give. I support clients in auditing their life and stress bucket as part of the work we do together. There are likely a lot of elements in your stress bucket that you cannot control, and often times life just gets heavy; but with every single one of my clients, when we've gotten honest at unpacking and auditing their stress bucket, there are always things contributing to their load that are optional or no longer serve them. This might be activities on their calendar, beliefs in their mind, or lifestyle practices that are leaving them depleted and burnt out.

When it comes to stress, there are three main goals:

1. Goal #1 is to decrease the likelihood of long-term chronic stress.

2. Goal #2 is to be able to reset from stressful events more quickly by improving vagal tone and knowing how to push back against our body's stress response in real time.

3. Goal #3 is to increase our overall capacity for stress.

We will all experience both acute and chronic stress to varying degrees in our life. The key is to be aware and equipped with tools to minimize negative impacts. And the best tools to control stress are the ones that have a direct, hardwired line to our autonomic nervous system.

As much as our stress response is a biologically hardwired mechanism, we have another biologically hardwired mechanism that can push back against our stress response in real time through the healing power of the vagus nerve.

The next chapter will take you on a journey to better get to know the vagus nerve, its various branches throughout the body, and its influential role in both mental and physical health.

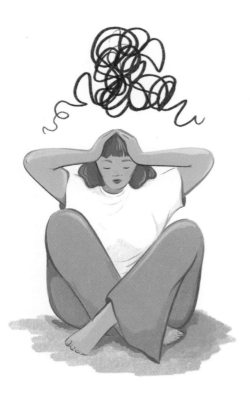

QUICK SUMMARY

- The autonomic nervous system is a constant seesaw between sympathetic activation and parasympathetic relaxation.

- Understanding this system and the different nervous system states empowers you to better work *with* the system to move toward healing instead of always feeling like they are working against you.

- The polyvagal theory and stress bucket analogy give working models to better understand and assess the nervous system in real time to know which tools are the right fit to move toward regulation.

- The interplay between sympathetic and parasympathetic activation turns the stress response on and off.

- Chronic and traumatic stress can wreak havoc on our psychology and physiology, decreasing our ability to feel safe and stay regulated. We also have an incredible capacity to heal and mitigate lasting effects through nervous system regulation.

- The vagus nerve makes up a huge part of our parasympathetic nervous system and holds the key modulating stress, optimizing mind-body connection, improving physical well-being, and combating anxiety and depression.

2

THE VAGUS NERVE

Understanding the vagus nerve holds the key to working with your mind and body—instead of constantly feeling like it's working against you.

The vagus nerve is your mind-body superhighway, sending nonstop information from body to brain and brain to body. It is the main component of the parasympathetic nervous system and oversees many important bodily functions. It plays a role in stress, mood, immune response, digestion, heart rate, and several other autonomic functions. If in chapter 1 you nodded your head *yes* to multiple symptoms, there's a good chance that your vagus nerve is a common thread. To understand the importance of your vagus nerve and the role it plays in your health and well-being, it is important to learn what it does, why it matters, and how it relates to your mental and physical health.

WHAT IS THE VAGUS NERVE?

The word *vagus* comes from the Latin word for "wandering" and is sometimes referred to as the "wandering nerve" because of the long and winding path it takes throughout most of the body. As the longest cranial nerve, the vagus nerve has both a left and a right side, traveling down the right and left sides of your body, from the brainstem to the colon, and is connected to the heart, lungs, gut, and other vital internal organs. It helps regulate the autonomic nervous system and its basic functions, like breathing, heart rate, blood pressure, hormones, and digestion. Imagine a tree with the most intricate root system you can imagine pulled out of the ground. (You would be blown away by how huge it is!)

The vagus nerve has both sensory and motor functions; sensory nerves carry signals from sensory organs to your brain to help you touch, taste, smell, and see, and motor nerves carry signals to your muscles or glands to help you move and function. The vagus nerve makes up 75 to 80 percent of your parasympathetic nervous system, regulating the fight, flight, or freeze responses that affect anxiety and your ability to handle emotional and physical stressors.

The vagus nerve connects vital internal organs, acting as a messenger. Its different branches send data from around the body to the brain, and instructions from the brain to the body.

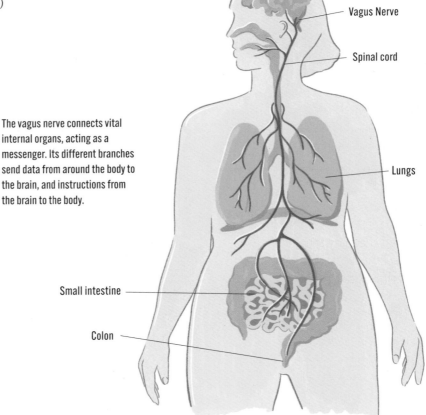

- Brain
- Vagus Nerve
- Spinal cord
- Lungs
- Small intestine
- Colon

VAGUS NERVE ANATOMY AND FUNCTION

There are various branches of the vagus nerve passing through your neck, chest, heart, lungs, abdomen, and digestive tract. They are constantly collecting and analyzing information that tells your brain what's going on in the body, and your brain then sends instructions back down. Understanding these different branches will help you better understand why certain practices I'll introduce you to later in this book are so effective at activating the vagus nerve. Let's start at the top of the vagus nerve and follow its course down through some of the primary pathways and branches.

KEEP THIS IN MIND AS YOU READ:

Functions of the vagus nerve are vast, and there are still many functions that neuroscientists and other researchers don't fully understand or know about yet. Still, there's much we do know, including the important fact that the vagus nerve makes up 75 to 80 percent of the parasympathetic nervous system. With so many parasympathetic nerve fibers, the vagus nerve plays an important role in helping you turn off or dampen your fight-or-flight response.

Researchers have also found that vagus nerve cells are 80 percent afferent, meaning they send information and instructions from the body to the brain, and just 20 percent efferent, meaning the communication comes from the brain to the body. When I talk about the mind-body connection, it's helpful to know that a majority of that conversation is happening *from the body to the brain*. Our physiology greatly impacts our psychology, which is why traditional top-down methods, like talk therapy or mindset work, fall short for many people struggling with chronic stress, anxiety, PTSD, or depression. With 80 percent of the conversation coming from the body, it's important to incorporate bottom-up, body-based practices, and vagus nerve healing is part of the approach to overall healing. Learning to understand and improve vagal health can play an important role in rebalancing the nervous system and decreasing many of the negative effects of chronic stress.

The Brainstem Connection

The vagus nerve originates in the medulla oblongata of the brainstem and consists primarily of four different types of nuclei that control specific nerve fibers, functions, and different types of information the vagus nerve carries. These nuclei are:

- **Dorsal motor nucleus:** This sends signals to help calm, regulate, and optimize various bodily functions, particularly in the lungs and intestines.

- **Solitary nucleus:** This sends sensory information from internal organs such as the lungs, heart, liver, spleen, gallbladder, pancreas, stomach, and intestinal tract and also receives afferent taste sensations from the tongue.

- **Spinal trigeminal nucleus:** This sends information about touch, pain, and temperature, including sensory information from specific parts of the ear, which will come into play with an ear massage tool you learn later in the book.

- **Nucleus ambiguous:** This sends out neurons with motor functions, specifically working muscles in the throat and upper airway, which I will later discuss activating with tools like gargling and humming. The nucleus ambiguous also contains some parasympathetic fibers that travel to the heart.

The Head and Neck

From the brainstem, various innervating branches of the vagus nerve run through the head and neck before moving down to the rest of the body. In the head, the vagus nerve reaches the ears (auricular branch), face, and muscles at the base of the tongue and soft palate. It plays a role in eye contact, facial expressions, and even the ability to tune in to other people's voices. In the neck, the vagus nerve regulates motor functions controlling certain neck and throat muscles responsible for speech, voice pitch, gag reflex, and swallowing. When you massage certain parts of your ear, trigger your gag reflex, or vocalize, your vagus nerve is activated.

The Thorax

The thorax is the chest region of your body where the vagus nerve oversees the various organs and much of their function. These organs include:

- **Trachea:** The trachea is one of the structures involved in breathing; the vagus nerve plays a role in maintaining smooth breathing and reflexes like sneezing, gagging, and coughing.

- **Lower part of the esophagus:** The vagus nerve provides reflex relaxation in the lower esophagus to move food to the stomach via swallowing.

- **Lungs:** The vagus nerve helps regulate airflow in the lungs, the primary respiratory organ.

- **Heart**: The vagus nerve plays a role in regulating and maintaining heart rate and blood pressure.

The Respiratory System

How you breathe makes a big difference in how
you feel as well as your heart rate, blood pressure,
autonomic functions, and even dental health.
Breathwork has become a trendy tool and topic,
one I will talk more about later in chapter 6. For
now, I'll just say that although I believe some of the
claims made about breathwork can be overstated,
it's well supported by research that your breath is
one of the most powerful levers you can pull to
affect the sympathetic-parasympathetic seesaw.

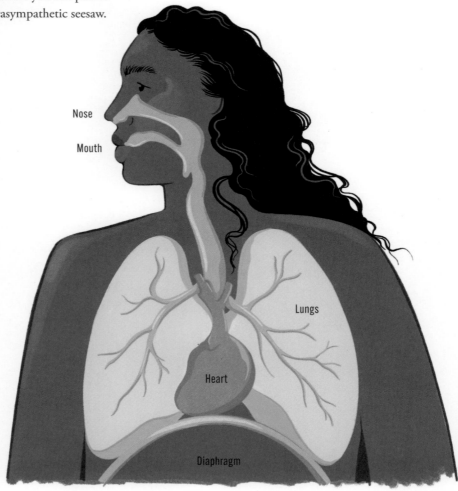

Let's look at some of the physiology behind that. How quickly and deeply you breathe, intentionally or unintentionally, increases or decreases your stress response, alters body chemistry, and impacts overall function via the vagus nerve. The vagus nerve connects neurons to one another, sending sensory information up to the brain, and the brain sends information back through motor pathways to change the way our organs are working. One of the best examples of this interplay happens through the respiratory system and translates into a tangible tool for decreasing our body's stress response.

Just below your lungs is a dome-shaped muscle called the diaphragm. When you inhale, the diaphragm flattens, pulling air into the lungs, and the chest cavity enlarges. When the chest cavity enlarges, your heart has a bit more room and expands as well. When the heart gets bigger, the rate of blood flow slows down, which sends a signal to the brain, and then the brain sends a signal back to speed up the heart to make sure there's regular blood flow. When you exhale, the diaphragm relaxes and returns to its domelike shape, pushing air out of the lungs. This re-shrinks the chest cavity and heart, increasing blood flow, which sends a signal to the brain, and the brain then sends a signal back to slow the heart down. So, when you inhale you are increasing your heart rate and when you exhale you are decreasing your heart rate; this is a natural balancing of the activating and relaxing mechanisms in the body.

When you inhale for five seconds, you're increasing your heart rate that entire time. When you exhale for five seconds, you're decreasing your heart rate that entire time. So, if you exhale longer than you inhale (known as extended exhale breathing), you can slow down your heart rate. This activates the parasympathetic relaxation response, allowing you to decrease and push back against stress in real time. Inversely, let's say you have to get a project done at work but you're feeling tired and struggling to focus. If you inhale longer or more intensely than you exhale, you will activate your sympathetic response. As long as you don't overdo it to the point of stress or anxiety, it could help give you the boost you need to wake up and focus.

The Abdomen

The organs of the abdomen are the final section of the body that the vagus nerve innervates. The abdominal branches of the vagus nerve start in the stomach, then move on to the liver, gallbladder, pancreas, spleen, intestines, and kidney. Again, I want to do a quick overview of some of the basic function of each of these organs so you can see how some seemingly unrelated symptoms may have the vagus nerve as a common thread.

- **Stomach:** When the body is in a relaxed state, the vagus nerve stimulates the stomach to function by releasing acid and regulating the smooth muscle cells to churn and push food from the stomach to your small intestines. When the vagus nerve is not working well and not sending these signals accurately or efficiently, it can lead to low stomach acid, causing problems in properly breaking down food. The vagus nerve also lets the brain know whether the gut is full or empty.

- **Liver:** The liver has many of functions that need input from the vagus nerve. Some of these influence or cause feelings of hunger, cravings for certain types of nutrients, bile production, balancing blood sugar, measuring fat intake, and filtering blood.

- **Gallbladder:** The gallbladder stores bile from the liver and then releases it into the first section of the small intestines to help the body break down fats from food. The pumping of the gallbladder sending bile into the digestive tract is mediated by the vagus nerve.

- **Pancreas:** The pancreas produces and releases insulin and glucagon to balance blood sugar levels. The vagus nerve sends signals to and from the pancreas and brain that optimize effectiveness of the digestive process and balance blood sugar levels.

- **Spleen:** The spleen fights invading germs in the blood, controls the level of blood cells (white blood cells, red blood cells, and platelets), and filters the blood to remove old or damaged red blood cells. When there's an infection, or something the body wants to fight off, the sympathetic branch activates inflammatory pathways; this is an instance in which inflammation is good and helpful. Once that job is done, the parasympathetic branch, via the vagus nerve, signals a halt to the inflammation process.

- **Intestines:** The intestines consists of the small intestines and the large intestines. The small intestines' main job is to break down and absorb macronutrients (carbohydrates, fats, and proteins). The vagus nerve regulates smooth muscle contractions that help move food through the small intestines. Then comes the large intestines, which is home to one of the most precious ecosystems in your body, the gut microbiome. The vagus nerve is the major pathway that relays information from our gut microbiome to our brain.

- **Kidneys:** You have two kidneys, one located on each side of your body. Their main jobs are to control blood pressure, cleanse the blood of toxins, and transform waste into urine. The vagus nerve controls several functions of the kidneys.

It's through these organs that the vagus nerve helps the brain and body modulate inflammation, regulate food intake and digestion, manage energy levels, maintain intestinal balance, manage blood sugar and blood pressure levels, and more.

THE GUT

There's been a great deal of discussion and research in the last decade on the mind-gut connection, and for good reason. The gut is often referred to as our "second brain" due to the magnitude of influence it has over so many other systems. The vagus nerve is the information highway that facilitates this mind-body conversation. To better understand this mind-gut connection, let's get more familiar with the gut.

What Is the Gut?

When I say the "gut," I am referring to the gastrointestinal system or digestive tract. It is made up of the mouth, salivary glands, esophagus, stomach, pancreas, liver, gallbladder, appendix, small intestines, large intestines, rectum, and anus. Most often when we refer to the "gut" it will be in reference to the microbiome and function of the intestines, but problems in any other part of the digestive tract can contribute to overall dysfunction. The gut, through digestion, breaks down the food we eat into nutrients and energy we need to live and thrive.

The saying "you are what you eat" is true in that what you consume becomes the foundation of each cell in your body. Food is used for brain and memory function; eye function; digestion and transportation of waste products; heart and blood health; repairing and strengthening bones, muscle, ligaments, tissues, and cells in the body; energy for mental and physical activities; and maintaining the immune system. The gut works to process and keep the contents within until it's safe for it to enter the bloodstream and the rest of the body.

The gut's jobs consist of the following:

- It sustains overall health and well-being.

- It absorbs, processes, and redistributes water and needed nutrients from what we consume.

- It produces and stores many neurotransmitters like serotonin and gamma-aminobutyric acid (GABA). Almost 90 percent of serotonin—a neurotransmitter that makes you feel happy, modulates pain perception, facilitates better sleep, and affects other functions vital to well-being—is produced in the gut.

- It is the primary player in maintaining the immune system.

- It modulates stress, mood, pain, and our general state of mind.

- It maintains your gut microbiome (see page 41).

- It communicates with the brain via the gut-brain axis (see page 41).

What Is the Gut Microbiome?

The gut microbiome is made up of trillions of microorganisms, including fungi and bacteria, in the intestines. Its role is to support immune function, control inflammation, digest and absorb nutrients, maintain energy production, and manage metabolism and weight, and it can also influence sleep and pain. A healthy gut microbiome has a plentiful and diverse microbial colony. A suboptimal gut microbiome has been linked to many health conditions, including anxiety, stress, depression, inflammatory bowel syndrome (IBS), fibromyalgia, chronic inflammation, food sensitivities, decreased immune function, complex pain, and even Alzheimer's disease. Ongoing research in this area is attempting to determine whether an unhealthy gut microbiome is the cause or result of some of these conditions, or to what extent it may be a bit of both. What is clear is that a healthy gut ensures health and well-being in numerous ways.

The gut-brain axis

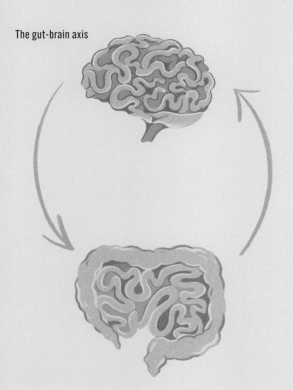

What Is the Gut-Brain Axis?

There is a constant bidirectional conversation happening between the brain and the gut. The "gut-brain axis" is a complex system that uses the vagus nerve as a communication highway to connect emotional and cognitive areas of the brain with overall gut function. Emotional signals from the brain play out in and influence the gut, and gut dysfunction can considerably influence the brain and our emotional state as well. It's common for people struggling with chronic stress, anxiety, or depression to also have digestive issues like IBS, constipation, or diarrhea, and vice versa; many people who struggle with digestive issues also have psychological symptoms.

Another thing worth noting is that common psychotropic drugs (antidepressants, antianxiety meditations, stimulants, antipsychotics, and mood stabilizers) have effects on both the brain and the gastrointestinal tract. Whether it's always negative or not is up for debate, though some studies show that antidepressants can reduce function and effectiveness of the gut microbiome. Everything likely comes with a give and take. The role of the gut-brain axis and the gut microbiome in relation to psychopharmacology still needs to be more comprehensively studied. Just be aware that it's all interconnected—taking a substance to change the state of your mind will likely influence other systems. Do your research and work with practitioners willing to educate and work with you in a flexible and personalized way.

If you want the big takeaway here, it's that the gut doesn't just help us digest our food; it also guides our emotions and psychological health. If you are someone who has symptoms in both arenas, there is likely a connection, so treating them separately may not be the best approach.

THE VAGUS NERVE AND MENTAL HEALTH

There are a number of things that contribute to mental health struggles, but the underlying impact of vagus nerve function and overall nervous system regulation cannot be emphasized enough. The following mental health categories I will touch on are ones I have personal and professional experience with. You may have a diagnosis or symptoms beyond this list, but I need to leave it to other books and practitioners because I don't have the personal or professional experience to cover them. I can say, though, that improving the overall function of your vagus nerve and autonomic nervous system has far-reaching beneficial effects.

Chronic Stress

Stress temporarily activates our sympathetic fight-or-flight response to meet the immediate threat of a stressor; afterward, our system resets. It becomes chronic stress or anxiety because of the inability of the vagus nerve to activate the parasympathetic response, thus keeping us in this fight-or-flight state.

At one point in my life, I was taking twenty-two graduate school credits, writing my master's thesis, working fifty-plus hours a week, taking care of a dog, overexercising, sleeping only five to six hours a night, and listening to some pretty nasty self-talk. I remember thinking to myself one night, "Someone busier than you is doing better than you." Oof, ouch. I had debilitating productivity-based self-worth that kept me spinning my wheels, constantly trying to do more and more and more. And this lasted for years.

What I learned was that chronic stress can come as a symptom of our choices or the reality of our life circumstances, but it's usually a mix of both. I created a life of chronic stress based on beliefs I acquired in my childhood and teenage years. You may have stressors in your life that are based on things like discrimination, poverty, natural disasters, or other situations entirely outside your control. It may not always be possible, at least not right now, to live a life with fewer stressors. The power in improving vagus nerve health is that it gives you the capacity to recover from your stress response faster and gives you tools to push back against that physiology in real time to dampen its impact. Stress isn't the problem; chronic stress is.

Daily modern life is full of layering stressors, big and small. Your sympathetic response is often activated by things like traffic, work responsibilities, relationships, processed foods, health concerns, systemic issues, or finances. If you don't have a way to turn off that activated stress response, the seemingly small stressors, combined with your larger ones, become chronic stress that wreaks havoc on your mind and body. The vagus nerve is the antidote to increasing your ability to manage and reset after stress via its major role in the parasympathetic state. When you learn to optimize

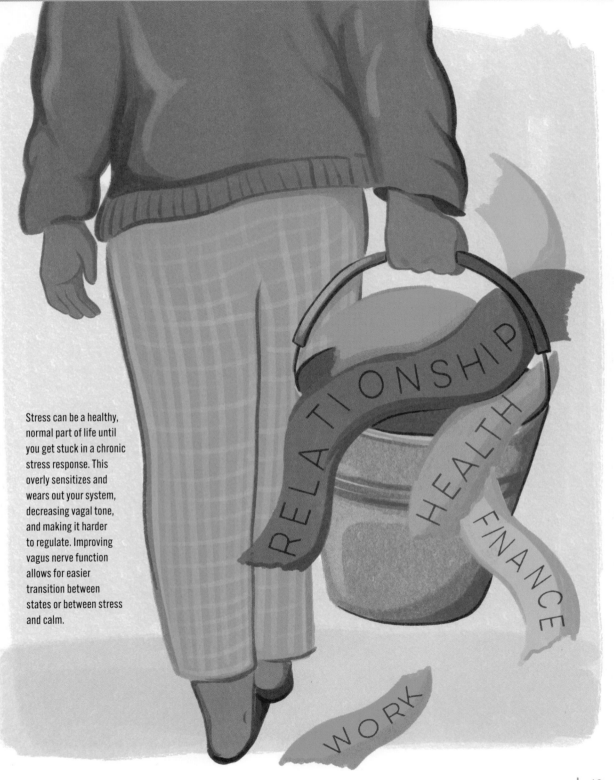

Stress can be a healthy, normal part of life until you get stuck in a chronic stress response. This overly sensitizes and wears out your system, decreasing vagal tone, and making it harder to regulate. Improving vagus nerve function allows for easier transition between states or between stress and calm.

and stimulate your vagus nerve with the tools and practices in this book (see practices in chapter 6), you will manage stress better and get better at resetting more quickly from stressful events, thus staying more regulated and present in whatever the situation is.

Remember the deadlift analogy I used in the introduction of this book? I often help my clients understand the balance between stress and carrying capacity by comparing it to a deadlift. For those who don't know, a deadlift is a common strength-training movement that usually involves a long barbell with weight on either side of the bar. The movement is to, with proper form, pick up the weighted bar from the floor. You wouldn't walk into a gym and expect to pick up a 300-pound bar without significant training. You also understand that if you tried to lift it anyway, there's a good chance you'll hurt yourself. Well, it's possible that you're currently doing the equivalent of lifting 300 pounds of stress. Your stressors outweigh your training, and it's hurting you. Of course you're struggling! No one trained or prepared you for the load life has handed you. When you can look at it this way, it's likely your symptoms begin to make more sense and a lot of the shame for not "handling your life better" can be let go.

Just like in the gym, we can manage this load better in two ways:

1. Make the load lighter.

2. Increase our capacity to carry the load.

Life naturally happens in seasons, some that feel heavier and others lighter. But if your daily life feels overwhelming, it's time to get honest about auditing your load. Take a look at what's in your stress bucket: What's on your calendar? How much clutter is in your home? What relationships in your life feel supportive versus draining? And then look at how you're supporting your basic biology that fuels your capacity to carry the load: How much sleep are you getting? What's the quality of your diet? How optimally do you breathe? How sedentary or active are you? And step into the work it takes to change some of those things.

As a person who has struggled with productivity-based self-worth for a lot of my life, I often carried around a load that was crushing. I said yes when I needed to say no. I took on more when I desperately shouldn't have and it took a very real toll on my mind and body. It was understanding the physiology of stress that finally helped me make some needed life changes to lighten my load and increase my capacity.

Working with your vagus nerve allows you to do both. In this book, you'll learn proactive and reactive practices that help you increase your stress threshold, enabling you to carry more. However, this same practice can also support you in decreasing the heaviness of what you're carrying. A healthy vagus nerve allows you to not only carry more but also to reset from stress much more quickly, helping to better balance that activation and relaxation seesaw.

Anxiety

You likely don't need a definition of anxiety. Instead, I want to help you reframe anxiety. Symptoms of anxiety are vast and different depending on who is experiencing them, but typically anxiety is a feeling of worry, fear, anticipation, or unease about something. Occasional anxiety is a normal part of life. It becomes an anxiety disorder when symptoms are excessive and interfere with day-to-day life. There are also physical symptoms of anxiety like fast heart rate, rapid breathing, sweating, or knots in your stomach. All of this is simply the by-product of being in a state of sympathetic activation. Anxiety in the moment carries an important message: It's telling you either "This is really important" or "This feels really familiar to a situation in which my sense of self or safety was threatened, so I need to pay attention to survive." So, what if we reframed our understanding of anxiety by substituting it with the word *activation*?

> "I feel really activated in social settings."

> "I struggle with overwhelming activation to the point of panic attacks."

> "I wake up feeling activated in the morning."

I often explain anxiety as an overestimation of threat paired with an underestimation of your ability to manage that threat. We often overestimate threat in the moment because our nervous system is on high alert. Your physiology drives your psychology, so when your body system is mobilized so is your brain. In an effort to keep you safe, you start to overthink, imagine worst-case-scenarios, and so on.

Activation isn't a problem (anxiety isn't a problem); a problem arises when these symptoms are excessive, disproportionate to the stressor at hand, or activated at the wrong time, when you are very much safe. What does this have to do with the vagus nerve? Great question.

Having a poorly functioning vagus nerve makes us more susceptible to stress and activation and less able to turn it off. When you internalize this reframe of seeing anxiety as activation, you will realize you aren't as helpless against it as you once felt. The tools and strategies you'll learn in this book will help you experience less anxiety over time and give you real-time tools that will help you push back against that sympathetic activation when you decide it's not needed to meet the situation at hand.

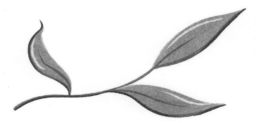

Depression

At one point I was told by medical professionals that depression was caused by a chemical imbalance in the brain. I've also been told that anxiety was hereditary and I should expect to take anxiety medications for years on end. These insufficient explanations and solutions are exactly what led me to the work I do with people today. Are neurotransmitters (chemicals) or genetics involved? You bet, but I believe it pays to dig deeper. There's a growing body of research disproving the chemical imbalance theory. Just because a drug that boosts your serotonin helps you feel better doesn't mean that some naturally occurring serotonin deficit is the cause of your symptoms. That's like saying that just because caffeine gives you more energy, it must be a lack of caffeine that's causing you to be tired. We understand that's simply not true.

What is likely contributing to you being exhausted is a combination of poor sleep, trauma, stress, not enough recreation time, and a need for more sunlight. Now, don't misunderstand this discussion to mean that I am in any way anti-medication: I'm absolutely not. There's a time and place for medication to be the right intervention for many people. It feels important to make another comment about this before moving on: Medication can also play a partial or temporary role. If your symptoms are so unmanageable that you're unable to take any other steps toward healing, then medication might help dampen those symptoms, giving you the capacity to take other healing steps. For many people, however, medication makes their symptoms worse or negatively impacts other body systems, like energy levels or digestion. When medication is the only solution offered, it often leaves people feeling hopeless.

The simple point I want to make is that medication is *AN* option, not *THE* option, and too often people are quickly offered this as a catchall solution to their symptoms. This robs them of the opportunity to dig

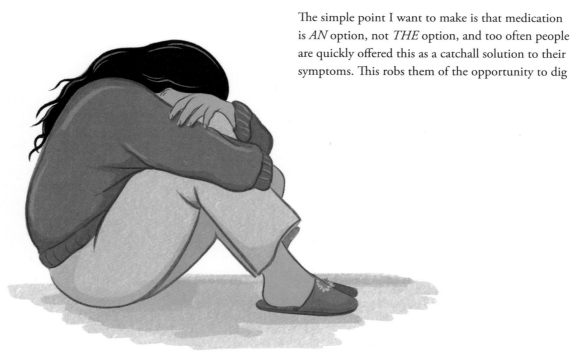

further down and heal at a deeper level. That deeper level for myself and hundreds of my clients has been to better understand their nervous system and how to work with it to move toward long-term healing.

Through the polyvagal theory, I learned that activity of the dorsal vagal branch of the vagus nerve creates many symptoms that we associate with depression, such as feelings of sadness, numbness, dissociation, hopelessness, worthlessness, guilt, and shame, along with other typical symptoms like loss in interest in things you once enjoyed, low mood, changes in eating habits, digestive issues, social isolation, and apathy. When helping clients understand depression through a nervous system lens, I often come back to the visual of the different nervous system zones. When the load on our nervous system gets too heavy, it pushes us down into the red zone (aka dorsal vagal shutdown). If anxiety is the warning, then depression is the shutdown. This is why prolonged anxiety begins to manifest as depression symptoms for so many people. Your nervous system has decided that it can't fight off or flee from the stressor, so the best chance at survival is to shut down.

Another reason this shutdown response might occur is if there was childhood trauma. Because fighting or running from a caregiver really wasn't an option, you instead disconnected or shut down and that pattern followed you to adulthood. The shutdown response is also common in the event of an assault by someone (or a system) bigger or stronger than you. This shutdown state that houses depression is an adaptive response to whatever has happened or is currently happening in your life. This state is your system saying that life is too painful for you to engage with, or it is too overwhelming and you don't have enough energy to engage with what is happening. This low-energy, low-feeling state has two priorities: to prevent further pain from being felt and/or to conserve energy.

I believe that the underlying problem for many is a lack of understanding our autonomic nervous system. In research, there is significant attention to the physiology of stress, but less so looking at the physiology of depression. When clients have come to me with a depression diagnosis, my approach is always multifaceted and personalized. But the foundation of our work is built on helping them understand and regulate their nervous system, part of which is working to improve the functioning of their vagus nerve.

Trauma

When we experience or witness distressing events, it leaves a lasting imprint on the mind and body. When you think of the word *trauma* you likely think of things like abuse, car accidents, or war. Those are traumatic, but so are things like school bullying, emotionally immature parents, poverty, discrimination, and lack of social interactions. Trauma can be the things that happened *to* you or the things that should have happened *for* you that didn't. It comes as a result of anything that challenged your felt sense of self or safety. (This often happens in situations where you lack a significant sense of context, choice, or connection.) Trauma can result from anything that happened too soon, too often, or too intensely. It comes from any experience or event that went beyond your coping skills and overwhelmed your nervous system, preventing you from fully completing a natural stress cycle. When this happens, the excess survival energy gets stored in the body, which often locks your system into a state of fight, flight, freeze, or shutdown. From a physiological standpoint, trauma is a buildup of stored survival stress in the body.

It's also important to note that trauma isn't universal; it isn't *what* happened but instead *how* you experienced it. In other words, it isn't the event, but instead what happened in your body, within your nervous system, during and after that event. What might be a normal Tuesday for an ER nurse or someone from a marginalized population might be the most traumatic thing you've ever experienced. Again, trauma is not universal. It becomes traumatic to you when you are unable to reset into a felt sense of safety.

Your vagus nerve is actively involved in your emotional well-being and can determine how much you are emotionally affected by a traumatic event, even long after it is over. Trauma is typically part of the story for those struggling with anxiety or depression because it rewrites our sense of self and safety, leading us to react accordingly to life. Hypervigilance, an elevated state of constantly assessing potential threats around you, is often the result of trauma. The anticipation of worst-case scenarios keeps our system constantly in sympathetic overdrive. Continued exposure to threats or traumatic situations can create lower heart rate variability, a way we measure the function of our vagus nerve. Low heart rate variability has been found to be associated with higher emotional sensitivity and impaired emotional regulation ability, and vice versa. High heart rate variability (indicating high vagus nerve function) is a marker that your body has an increased capacity for stress and emotional regulation, making it less likely that a stressful situation gets stored as trauma in your body.

Another thing to note in relation to the vagus nerve and trauma is the topic of social connection. Safe and authentic social connection activates your vagus nerve, increasing your parasympathetic response and sense of safety. There is valuable research showing that the likelihood of something being registered and stored as trauma can be significantly reduced if you have quick access to regulating social connection. For example, if you and I were both sitting in the back of the same car while it was in an accident, our experience of that event in the moment might be similar, but it's impact could vary significantly.

If you went home to a partner who was able to help you process and calm down from the experience, but I rushed into work or returned home to an empty apartment with no one to co-regulate with, the likelihood of that event having a negative and lasting imprint is much higher for me than for you. Of course, other things are at play, such as past experiences and current vagus nerve health. The point I'm hoping to drive home is that as humans we are hardwired for connection, and the deprivation of such can be traumatic in and of itself. On the other hand, the cultivation of positive social connections activates the vagus nerve and can act as a protector against trauma.

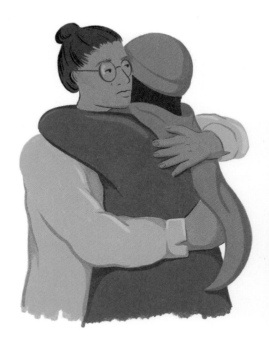

ADHD

My professional expertise is in addressing anxiety and depression, but my personal experience has also included attention deficit hyperactivity disorder (ADHD). So, while discussing ADHD I'm inviting you, more or less, into the inner musings and journey of my personal experience. As with everything in this book, take what serves you and move on from what does not.

I was diagnosed with ADHD after a simple questionnaire in a psychiatrist's office (it took about ten minutes). Do I think the diagnosis was accurate? Probably. But was it the entire picture? No, it was not. Remember when we were talking about chronic stress and I shared with you that laundry list of things I was involved in all at the same time? This was about the time in my life I was diagnosed with ADHD. I was prescribed medication that was really helpful. It helped me focus enough to write that master's thesis, make some important work decisions, and get more done.

The problem is that the psychiatrist never asked me about my life. He never asked me how much sleep I was getting, how stressed I was feeling, or how much or little exercise I was doing. He didn't collect enough information to know whether these symptoms of inability to focus, irritability, excessive talking, impulsiveness, or forgetfulness were because of true ADHD or simply a result of chronic stress and nervous system dysregulation. I began to wonder whether this medication was actually something helping me manage ADHD symptoms or whether it was a substance that simply increased my capacity to facilitate an unsustainable lifestyle. I have come to the conclusion that it was both.

What's the difference between true ADHD and symptoms of chronic stress, trauma, or a dysregulated nervous system? The reality is the symptoms can look the same but have very different root causes, thus leading to frequent misdiagnosis. Research to date has shown that ADHD has a strong hereditary component and can also be the result of significant head injuries, premature birth, or prenatal exposure to things like alcohol or nicotine. The only one of these, to my knowledge, that could apply to me would be a hereditary component, but even that I'm not entirely sure about, because there's also a lot of generational trauma in my bloodline.

After learning more and more about my nervous system in relation to my anxiety and depression, I got curious about its role in my ADHD. I decided, with the support of a doctor, to quit taking my ADHD medication entirely and instead focus on regulating my nervous system and decreasing the stressors in my life. It's been seven years since I took medication for my ADHD.

The conclusion I've come to is that, for me, both are true: I have what we label as ADHD *and* I just so happened to be living an incredibly dysregulated and unsustainable lifestyle when I got my diagnosis. Even with all the work I've done to improve my vagal tone and regulate my nervous system, my symptoms are not gone, but they are manageable. And in some cases, I've even begun to use them to my advantage. I'm lucky to be in a place where I have alternative tools, many that I'll be teaching you in this book, that have supported me doing things that require deep concentration (like writing a book!).

Bringing It All Together

Thanks for coming with me on that journey of the vagus nerve through the body. I hope you can now see how and why this nerve plays such a pivotal role in our well-being—and how it is often the common thread between what may seem like completely unrelated symptoms. The impact of the vagus nerve on human physiology is vast and significant, and it plays a huge role in our psychology as well. Low vagus nerve function impacts us physically, increasing risk for things like digestion issues, chronic pain, autoimmune conditions, and heart disease. It also impacts us psychologically, increasing risk for and symptoms of anxiety, PTSD, ADHD, and depression.

Many people are diagnosed with mental or physical health conditions in isolation and without considering that their problems might arise from dysfunction of their autonomic nervous system. It is my experience that helping a person regulate their nervous system, in large part by accessing the healing power of their vagus nerve, causes many of their symptoms to decrease or disappear. Yes, your results may vary. But I am optimistic you will be part of the majority of people who benefit from improved knowledge and health of the vagus nerve.

Now, it's one thing to understand all of this in theory; it's another thing entirely to personalize information about *the* nervous system to what it means for *your* nervous system. In the next chapter, I'll walk you through how to start exploring your nervous system to pave the way for your unique healing journey.

QUICK SUMMARY

- The vagus nerve is one of the most vital nerves of the human body. It not only connects multiple organs but also facilitates several vital processes that take place in the body.

- The various branches of the vagus nerve run from your brainstem down to your large intestines. Each branch contributes to vital sensory and motor functions.

- The vagus nerve makes up 75 to 80 percent of the parasympathetic nervous system, which helps dampen the fight-or-flight response and reset from stressful situations.

- About 80 percent of the mind-body conversations that happens through our vagus nerve superhighway is afferent, meaning messages from the body to the brain.

- Your vagus nerve is actively involved in your psychological well-being. Low heart rate variability, a measure for vagus nerve function, is associated with higher emotional sensitivity, impaired emotional regulation ability, and a decreased capacity for stress. Higher vagal health is associated with the opposite.

- The vagus nerve is a vital piece in unlocking overall wellness. It is one of the fastest ways we can optimize our physiology to positively influence our psychology.

3

EXPLORING YOUR UNIQUE NERVOUS SYSTEM

Nervous system regulation begins with awareness. The greater the awareness, the greater your potential to reconnect to your body, rewire your mind, and reclaim your life.

It is helpful to understand how your nervous system and vagus nerve work in general, but what is even more powerful is to explore and understand how that applies uniquely to you, which is exactly what we will be exploring together in this chapter.

In chapter 1 you got an overview of the autonomic nervous system and the different states or zones. Chapter 2 took you on a journey through the body to understand the powerful influence the vagus nerve has on this system and on your overall well-being. The vagus nerve is important physiology, but instead of creating a mindset around trying to *hack your vagus nerve* as a way to heal, I want to help you understand and build a relationship with your whole nervous system—and then help you leverage one of the most powerful parts of that system, the vagus nerve.

The goal of this chapter is to take the broad education you just received and make it personal to you. I'll guide you through exploring the unique ways in which you experience each nervous state and help you discover where your current baseline is set. This will provide a framework for more personalized application of the tools you'll soon learn.

TUNING IN WITH INTEROCEPTION

Have you ever felt your stomach growling? Your heart pounding? Your eyes growing heavy? Or butterflies in your stomach? You notice these sensations in your body with the help of an important sense: interoception.

Interoception is the sense that enables you to be aware of and understand internal sensations and signals from the body. This could be fairly obvious things like hunger, thirst, exhaustion, or pain, or the more subtle differences in how you somatically experience being excited versus anxious or calm versus shut down. Interoception is like your sixth sense, providing you with information about your internal body state that is separate from the traditional five senses of sight, hearing, touch, taste, and smell. This sense is a really big deal and has a huge influence on many areas of your life, including self-regulation, mental and physical health, and social connection. So how exactly does it work?

This sense is at work all the time, monitoring your entire body—heart, lungs, stomach, bladder, muscles, skin, eyes, and more—collecting information about how these parts of your body *feel*. This information is then sent to the brain to help you identify how you feel or what you need. For example, does your stomach feel empty, full, gassy, tingly, or something else? Is your heart rate slow and steady or racing? Then, your brain uses this information about how your body feels and is functioning to clue you in on your physiological needs or emotions: Are you hungry? Nervous? Tired? Sad?

At the most basic level, interoception helps us answer the question "How do I feel?" in any given moment and is a vital aspect of self-awareness and self-regulation. Having clear awareness of your body signals gives you important feedback about how you are feeling and valuable information about the situation at hand that can help you take appropriate action.

For example, if your stomach is growling, it signals that you are hungry, which then motivates you to take action to eat. But if you're feeling knots in your stomach, this may clue you in on the fact that you're feeling nervous or anxious, which urges you to seek support, self-regulate, or move away from that particular situation. Interoception serves as your motivation to self-regulate in a way that restores a sense of comfort and safety within your body (given that you have the tools and resources to do so, again, something I hope you'll get from this book).

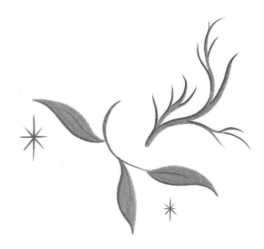

LET'S DO A QUICK INTEROCEPTION REFLECTION:

- How connected to and aware of your body signals are you currently?

- How aware are you of physiological sensations that cue hunger, fullness, thirst, pain, and sleep?

- Do you pursue activities that bring you comfort and regulation?

- Do you avoid activities that consistently dysregulate you?

- For the following questions insert any feeling or sensation ((e.g., calm/anxious/hungry/angry).

- How does your body feel when it is calm/anxious/angry/hungry (or any other emotion or physiological cue)?

  - How do you know when you are _____?
  - What makes you feel _____?
  - How does your body feel different when you are a little _____ versus really _____?
  - Are you able to notice these sensations early, maybe when they are slowly building, or only when they feel big and intense?

- Was it easy to answer those questions, or did it take some thought?

If you had a clear answer to a majority of the questions above, then your interoception skills are more fine-tuned. If you answered "no" or "I don't know" to some of those questions, you're likely a bit disconnected from your body cues and what they mean. And if the latter is true, don't worry, you're not alone! The fast-paced and busy nature of most our lives keeps us trapped in our head, just jumping from one thing to the next. Research has made it abundantly clear that interoception can be improved through various mindfulness practices and other engaging activities that help people explore and understand their own inner experiences.

Cultivating interoception is a practice of intentionally inviting yourself into connection and communication with your body and nervous system—a big reason you probably made your way to a book like this! Every time you intentionally tune in and check in with your body sensations, you improve interoception. Do this often enough and, over time, it will become something that happens much more automatically and intuitively.

All of this is vital when it comes to nervous system regulation, because different tools are needed to regulate depending on which nervous system state you're in. In a moment I'll walk you through mapping out your nervous system and exploring how you uniquely experience the three primary nervous system states of regulation, activation, and shutdown. This practice is the start of creating a clearer map of how to work with your nervous system in an effective way.

NERVOUS SYSTEM MAPPING

Mapping your nervous system is a practice in which you explore how you uniquely experience each of the nervous system states so that you can more quickly identify when you are in states of dysregulation and access the tools that help you shift toward regulation. In each state you'll try to identify the different sensations, emotions, thoughts, and behaviors that are specific to that state.

Here's a quick reminder of the three primary nervous system states and an overview of what is commonly experienced in each.

REGULATION
(Ventral Vagal)

This is your regulated state of safety, presence, and connection. Here are some common ways you might experience this state:

SENSATIONS	EMOTIONS	THOUGHTS	BEHAVIORS
Steady	Calm	"I can."	Check in with yourself before making decisions
Relaxed	Connected	"There's enough time."	Connect to self and others
Grounded	Curious	"I am capable and able do this."	Act with intention and purpose
Present	Safe	"I can cope."	Have joyful sexuality and intimacy
Focused	Happy	"Everything is okay."	Are curious and flexible in communication and situations
Energized but not overstimulated	Present	"I'm enjoying this."	Take breaks or rest when wanted or needed without guilt
Overall your body feels just right	Creative		
	Content		
	Desirous		
	Open		

ACTIVATION
(Sympathetic)

This is your self-protective, hyperaroused state of dysregulation, often referred to as your fight-or-flight response. Your nervous system sends you here when it decides there is danger and there's something you can do to get away from it or make it stop; therefore, this state is all about taking action—it is a state of mobilization. Here are some common ways you might experience this state:

SENSATIONS	EMOTIONS	THOUGHTS	BEHAVIORS
Rapid heartbeat	Concerned	"I must do this now."	Have a hard time relaxing or slowing down
Shallow or fast breathing	Confused	"It has to be done just right or else ..."	Need to control things
Sweaty or clammy palms	Annoyed	"If I slow down everything will fall apart."	Overwork
Tight chest	Irritated	"Are they mad at me?"	Don't take breaks
Muscle tension	Worried	"There is not enough time!"	Always on the go
Clenching	Anxiety	"I have to fix this."	Trouble sleeping
Heighted alertness of all senses	Anger	Constantly thinking about worst-case scenarios	Fidgety, nail biting, pacing
Shaking	Rage		Thoughts always racing, easily distracted
Tunnel vision	Panic		
Dizziness	Urgency		
Urgency or need to move	Out of control		
Body heat	Too much		
Fidgety			

SHUTDOWN
(Dorsal Vagal)

This is your self-protective, hypoaroused state of dysregulation. Your nervous system sends you here when it decides there is stress or danger that feels overwhelming and outside your ability to cope in any way. This often happens when the stress is too big, happens too often, or lasts too long. This state helps you conserve energy and leave your body so that you don't have to feel the perpetual pain of what is occurring. It is a state of immobilization and shutdown. Here are some common ways you might experience this state:

SENSATIONS	EMOTIONS	THOUGHTS	BEHAVIORS
Numb	Apathy	"I can't."	Isolating, withdrawing from people or activities you used to enjoy
Disconnected	Disconnected	"It doesn't even matter."	Staying in bed
Distant	Depressed	"I don't matter."	Difficulty speaking up or making eye contact
Blank	Numb	"Nothing will ever change."	Body doesn't want to move
Heavy	Out of it	"No one cares."	Flat facial expressions or tone of voice
Cold	Dissociated	"What's the point?"	Difficulty focusing
Limp	Hopeless	"Everything is too hard."	
Low energy	Helpless	"I just want to go to sleep so it goes away."	
Foggy	Shut down	"I'm all alone."	
Slow and shallow breathing	Feeling incapable	"I'm invisible and unlovable."	
Not being in body	Disinterested		
Exhaustion	Lonely		
Fatigue			

Each nervous system state has general characteristics that are universal. Broadly understanding each state simply paves the way for you to create a personal nervous system map exploring the unique ways in which you experience, feel, think, and act in each of these different states.

Mapping *Your* Nervous System

What I just shared with you was a general mapping of these three states. The next step is to create a nervous system map that is personal to *you*. Taking the time to cultivate this awareness is what helps strengthen interoception and enables you to regulate more effectively. The goal of this is to be able, in any given moment, to confidently answer these fundamental nervous system regulation questions:

1. Which nervous system state am I in right now?

2. How do I know that I am in that state?

3. Do I want to do something to change that? If so, what?

To create a map of your unique nervous system, make a similar chart to the one on pages 56 and 57. Then take time to go through each of the nervous system states and explore how you uniquely experience these four categories, asking yourself these questions:

- **Sensations:** What does it feel like in my body when I'm in this state? What color, temperature, or texture does this state feel like?

- **Emotions:** What emotions do I experience when I'm in this state?

- **Thoughts:** What thoughts do I have when I'm in this state? When I'm in this state, how would I finish this sentence: "The world is . . ." or "I am . . ."

- **Behaviors:** What actions do I take, or not take, when I'm in this state? What does my sleep/eating/substance/technology use look like when I'm in this state?

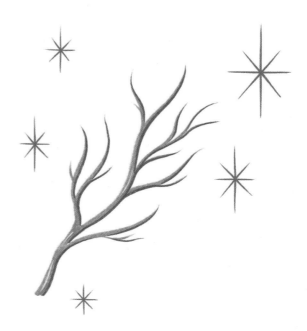

Now fill out what you currently have awareness of—though know that this will get more detailed and clear as time goes on. As you begin to mindfully pay attention to your nervous system in real time, you'll become more aware of the subtle shifts and things that show up for you in each state. As you notice more, I encourage you to add that to your profile map. This helps you more confidently know which state you're in, catch yourself slipping into dysregulation earlier, and course correct sooner. This is also crucial awareness to have as you start to explore and experiment with different nervous system regulation tools because different tools work for the different nervous system states. What works to help you feel less anxious is likely something different than will help you feel less depressed or angry. And whenever you're using a new tool, it's helpful to do a process of assess, use the tool, and reassess. You'll first check in and see how you're feeling, practice the tool, and then check in again to see whether there were any changes in how you felt. This process will help you identify the regulation tools that are the most helpful for you.

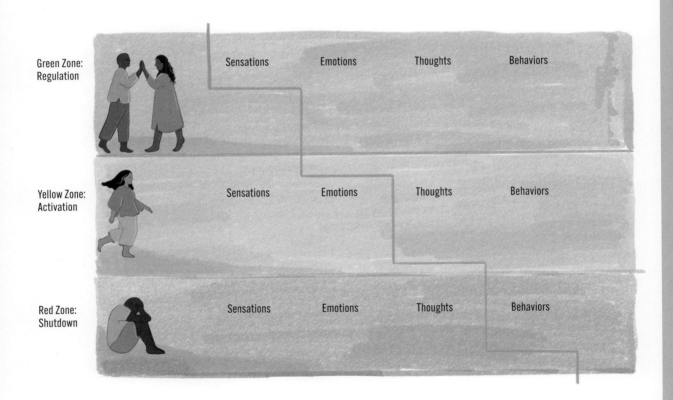

Green Zone:
Regulation

Sensations   Emotions   Thoughts   Behaviors

Yellow Zone:
Activation

Sensations   Emotions   Thoughts   Behaviors

Red Zone:
Shutdown

Sensations   Emotions   Thoughts   Behaviors

IDENTIFYING YOUR BASELINE STATE

In addition to mapping and becoming familiar with how you experience each of the nervous system states, it is helpful to pause and identify where you land most often, what I call your current baseline or default state.

Do you default to being more activated, anxious, and reactive?

Like my client Michelle (see page 26), who often felt reactive and anxious, do you feel like you're quick to instinctively react instead of intentionally respond? Do you find yourself overthinking or planning for worst-case scenarios? Do you lose it over the tiniest things sometimes? (You may logically know you're overreacting, but you can't seem to help it.) Is it hard for you to sit still? Do you feel like your heart is always racing? Do you have a running to-do list of a million things that all feel urgent? Do you clench your jaw or hold a lot of tension elsewhere in your body? Do your emotions feel big and hard to control? These can all be signs that you spend most of your time in sympathetic activation, or the "yellow zone" (see page 57).

Are you shut down, depressed, and flat?

One of my clients explained this to me as hitting rock bottom but getting kind of comfortable there. They obviously didn't want to stay there, yet this low state had become so familiar and robbed them of so much energy and motivation that it sometimes didn't feel worth it to try to climb their way out. Do you feel overwhelmed to the point of shutting down? Do you feel like you want to do things but find yourself frozen and unable to? Do things you used to enjoy not sound fun anymore? Do you have an urge to stay in bed, isolate, and not go anywhere or do anything? Do you often wonder "what's the point" or think "it doesn't even matter?" These can all be signs that you're stuck in dorsal vagal shutdown, or the "red zone" (see page 57).

Are you regulated, content, and grounded?

This is likely what you're hoping to experience more often and eventually cultivate as your default state. You feel calm, present, and safe. Even if things aren't going your way, you feel capable and able to handle the situation. In this state, you're able to feel playful, curious, creative, and collaborative. You connect authentically with people around you and feel like you have purpose. These can all be signs that you're settled into a state of parasympathetic regulation, or the "green zone" (see page 56).

Which nervous system state feels the most familiar to you? Remember to explore this from a place of curiosity and not judgment. There's no right or wrong current baseline. You're simply trying to gather information so that you can set a clearer path forward if you'd like something different. Understanding where you default to is helpful in informing the types of regulation tools and practices that might be most regulating for you.

GETTING TO "OF COURSE"

When my clients are trying to better understand their nervous system and symptoms, I invite them to think about the current state of their nervous system in terms of this equation:

Current state of your nervous system

=

Past lived experience

+

Current life circumstances

–

Coping skills/resourcing

This can refer to any specific moment or in looking at your overall baseline. I've found that laying it out like a math equation takes a lot of judgment out. Remember, your nervous system is always working for you in the only way it knows how based on your biological hardwiring and your past lived experiences. When you take time to pause and step back, you'll find that all your symptoms make sense through this nervous system lens.

Let's take a quick look at some recent conversations I've had with clients where they were able to use this new framework to see certain situations differently. Note: For privacy, I have changed the names of my clients.

Making Sense of Stress at Home

Jane is a stay-at-home mom of three. She came into a session frustrated that she is always irritated with her kids, often finds herself yelling, and feels like a bad mom overall. Together we began collecting the pieces of this equation to help her understand all of this through a nervous system lens.

Growing up, her mom yelled often, and her dad wasn't helpful with any of the kid or house duties, so even though she's married to a partner who is totally willing to help out she has a hard time asking for support. During the day she rarely gets a break; it's just one thing after another after another. She feels overstimulated and disrespected when the kids don't listen and that often leads to her yelling. She hates when she yells, but she feels like it just happens, and the truth is, it often works for getting her kids to listen, but she still feels guilty and wants to stop.

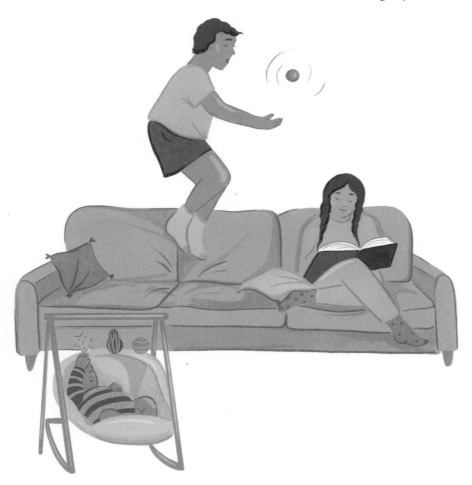

PAST LIVED EXPERIENCE:

Mom who yelled, dad who wasn't available for or willing to offer mom support, didn't feel heard as a child

+

Current life circumstances: Three age-appropriately chaotic and boundary-pushing kids, overstimulation, belief that she can't take a break or ask for support

-

Coping skills/resourcing: Sitting outside helps her but she rarely does it and she couldn't identify any other tools she has to feel less stressed

=

Current state of her nervous system:
Activated, leaving her quick to be reactive and anxious

Once we talked through that nervous system equation, she took a noticeable deep breath and shared, "I get it. I'm overstimulated and feel unsupported (even though I'm not), which is making me really activated; of course I yell. I don't feel like anyone is listening to me, I didn't feel heard much as a kid either, and yelling is what was modeled for me growing up. My brain also has a lot of evidence that it's what works on my kids too, even though I logically don't believe it's the only thing that could work. I just can't get myself to a place where I think I have any other option. My nervous system just knows it can't take anymore, my kids need to listen or I'll die, so I yell."

Looking at this, it makes sense, she makes sense, her feelings make sense, her actions *all make sense*. It's just hard to see that sometimes when you're in the thick of it. You can logically know better and still not have the capacity to do better when you're operating from survival mode. The reality is that your nervous system really doesn't know the difference between the stress brought on by noisy kids versus a tiger; all it knows is that you better fight, flee, or shut down from this threat if you want to live. Yelling is the only way she currently knows how to minimize that threat (get her kids to stop fighting or yelling or clean up, etc.) and so that's what she does—*of course* she does.

Understanding Why You Hold Back at Work

My client Julie shared that in work meetings when a coworker would push back against what her boss was saying she would think things like, "Oh no, they're going to get in trouble, they shouldn't push back or speak up like that." And then she would watch the person not get in trouble, or even if he did, he still stood by his objections.

Eventually, she came to be envious of her coworker's ability to speak up and be confident when she so often found herself shutting down anytime feedback was given and just going along with things she didn't agree with. After some coaching, she was able to lay it out in a similar equation:

PAST LIVED EXPERIENCE:

Her mom taught her that self-sacrifice was just what you did, and her needs came second to those around her. She also went to a private Catholic school, where the teachers often shamed and punished anyone who spoke up.

+

Current life circumstances: In a male-dominated field, is often spoken over, doesn't push back or ask for what she wants

-

Coping skills/resourcing: On the drive home she will often cry or just push it all away

=

Current state of her nervous system:
Almost always anxious and quick to shut down, constantly on the edge between the yellow and red zones

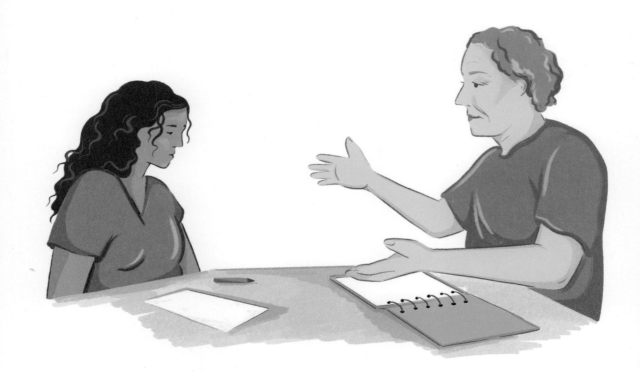

When I asked Julie why she thinks she shuts down versus her coworker who speaks up and doesn't seem to be bothered by the conflict, her first response was, "Well, because I'm just a pushover." After going through the equation with her, I asked again, and it was clear to her that the reason her coworker spoke up so easily and she couldn't was because their equations looked very different. His past lived experiences + current life circumstance created a very different reality for him than it did for her.

Maybe he was even on the debate team in high school, so not only was conflict or presenting contrary ideas practiced, but it was also encouraged. Maybe he was praised for being the loudest in the room. Or maybe his home life wasn't great and he had to learn to be the biggest and loudest to keep himself safe. Or maybe he's done a considerable amount of his own healing work to manage feelings of discomfort about

speaking up and can do so now when it feels important to him. He's also a male in a male-dominated field, which provides a different experience than often being the only female in a room. The specifics of his equation aren't relevant other than to add context to understanding that the way we show up in the world in any given moment always makes sense based on these components. Suddenly her narrative shifted from "Something is wrong with me" to "Oh, of course it makes sense."

Of course she doesn't push back or speak up; that doesn't feel safe to her nervous system. *Of course* she shuts down when feeling criticized because that's how she escaped the perpetuated emotional pain of being criticized at home and in school. *Of course* she thinks she's the problem or not good enough because that messaging was so readily available growing up.

The Power of "Of Course"

"Of course" has become some of the most powerful words used when working with clients. "Of course" is the internal shift from "something is wrong with me" to "I get it, it makes sense, now what?" It can create a shift from feeling like you need to heal because you're broken to instead wanting to heal because you simply want something different for yourself and your life. The old programming of how to show up and react in certain situations doesn't match what you really need to stay safe or what you really want to feel like.

This reframe and new understanding is what happens when you take the time to cultivate nervous system awareness, not just in general but in the context of how it uniquely plays a role in your life. This shift in understanding provides a powerful reframe for why you behave, feel, or act the way you do—because it's simply how you've been programmed to behave, feel, or act in these types of situations.

There's a powerful shift that occurs when you move from thinking, "I'm broken, I suck, this just is the way it is" to "Oh, it makes sense that I react or feel this way *and* I'd still like to change it." Put another way: *You are just a bigger version of the child that had to come up with a ton of creative ways to feel seen, heard, safe, and get your needs met.*

All of your symptoms, all of *you*, makes sense through this nervous system lens. By stepping back to explore your unique nervous system map and current nervous system baseline, you can start to move through your world and heal through self-compassion and curiosity instead of judgment and shame.

As I mentioned at the beginning of this chapter, it's not just about hacking your vagus nerve; it's about building a relationship with your entire nervous system *and then* understanding the powerful role that your vagus nerve plays in the overall health of that system.

Thanks for taking a step back with me in this chapter to explore the greater role your nervous system plays. In the next chapter, we will zoom back in on the vagus nerve to assess its current baseline before diving into all the tangible tools and lifestyle practices that will help you regulate your nervous system and access the healing power of your vagus nerve.

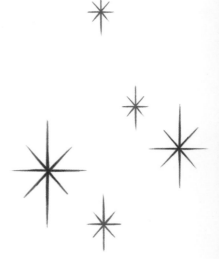

QUICK SUMMARY

- Interoception is the sense that enables you to be aware of and understand internal sensations and signals from the body. Cultivating interoception is a valuable part of nervous system regulation.

- Each nervous system state has a unique set of sensations, emotions, thoughts, and behaviors that come with it. Creating a nervous system map that is unique to you empowers you with the awareness to recognize which state you're in. Because different tools work better for different states, this provides a foundation for overall regulation.

- Three foundational nervous system regulation questions you want to be able to answer in any given moment are:

  1. Which nervous system state am I in right now?

  2. How do I know that I am in that state?

  3. Do I want to do something to change that? If so, what?

- Before trying to fix anything, you first need to get to a place of curiosity, understanding, and compassion for your current baseline and why you feel, think, and act the way you do based on your past lived experience, current life circumstances, and regulating tools you do or do not yet have. Changing the narrative from "There's something wrong with me that I have to fix" to "Oh, of course, this makes sense. Now what do I want instead?" is an important step in this healing work.

- Accessing the healing power of your vagus nerve starts by understanding the overall functioning of the nervous system it is a part of and the role that plays in your overall mental and physical well-being.

4

MEASURING VAGAL TONE

It's easier to meaningfully manage things that we can measure. Let's look at how to measure vagal tone.

Vagal tone is a measure of the activity and function of the vagus nerve. It can vary depending on several factors, which we will discuss in this chapter. High vagal tone is a good thing and refers to a state in which the vagus nerve is active and functioning properly—sending signals to the body's organs and systems in a way that promotes balance and overall well-being. This correlates with having better emotional regulation, stable energy, higher stress tolerance, good digestion, and improved mental and physical health. Low vagal tone refers to a state in which the vagus nerve is not active or functioning properly. It's not sending signals to the body in an effective or efficient way, which can contribute to a variety of symptoms and conditions. You may notice things like poor stress management, increased reactivity, hormone imbalances, digestive issues, anxiety, depression, and other negative mental and physical health symptoms.

It's important to note that high or low vagal tone is a relative term and unique to individuals. The most important thing to know is that vagal tone is adaptable and, regardless of where you are right now, it can improve and have a profound impact on your mental and physical health.

HIGH VERSUS LOW VAGAL TONE

For the purposes of understanding vagal tone, think about the vagus nerve like a muscle. A muscle with *lower tone* is weaker and less functional that a muscle with *higher tone*, which we understand as being stronger and therefore more capable. It's not a perfect analogy, but you get the idea. And just like there's a lot we've studied about muscle tone, there's a lot we've learned about what happens as a result of having low versus high vagal tone.

Vagal tone plays a pivotal role in well-being. You know this by now, but there are specific things we see that correlate with low versus high vagal tone. I have three hopes in laying out this side-by-side chart on the next page comparing low versus high vagal tone.

- First, I hope that you will quickly identify more with one column than the other. If you find yourself familiar with many of the symptoms in the low vagal tone column, refrain from layering any judgment onto this. For now, it's not a good or bad thing; it's simply information and you get to decide what to do about it.

- Second, I hope that nodding yes to many symptoms in a particular column will help you find and understand a common thread between some seemingly unrelated symptoms you struggle with.

- And third, I hope that seeing the mental and physical benefits of having higher vagal tone can act as a compassionate—and research-supported—invitation to take improving vagal tone seriously for your overall wellness. I know it did for me.

As I've prioritized better understanding my vagus nerve, minimizing things that lower tone, and intentionally building in practices that improve vagal tone, my overall well-being has increased. I'm a mom, wife, coach, business owner, author, podcast host, and real-life human and all that comes with it. Being more resilient toward stress, being able to make decisions more quickly, having improved immunity, and all the things you see in the chart have made moving through my daily life and balancing all those things much more manageable, and most of the time even enjoyable. I have better emotional regulation, I bounce back from stressful situations more quickly, my digestive issues have cleared up, I have more energy, and I have a healthy physiological baseline—decreasing my overall stress response—in a way that has supported me in much of my deeper trauma healing journey.

Let me be clear: Improving your vagal tone is not the magic ticket to solving all of life's problems. My personal healing journey and the work I do with clients is integrative and multifaceted, involving many different healing modalities. However, what lies as the foundation to and at the center of all of them is the nervous system, and your vagal tone is central to the overall functioning of that system. Let's take a look first at what sometimes can go wrong or cause low vagal tone.

	Low Vagal Tone May Be a Factor In . . .	High Vagal Tone May Lead To . . .
Heart Rate Variability (HRV)	Lower HRV, which is an indicator of poorer cardiovascular health (e.g., hypertension) and nervous system dysregulation	Higher HRV, which is an indicator of good cardiovascular health and a resilient nervous system
Emotional Regulation	Anxiety, depression, and emotional reactivity because you are less able to reset efficiently after stressful situations	Better emotional regulation and stress tolerance, which can lead to a greater sense of well-being and reduction in risk of mood disorders like anxiety and depression
Cognitive Function	Cognitive impairment, memory loss, or difficulty concentrating	Improved memory, attention, and decision making
Energy Levels	Feelings of fatigue and tiredness throughout the day	More sustained and predictable energy levels
Inflammation	Higher inflammation throughout the body, which can increase risk of chronic illness	Lower inflammation throughout the body, which can reduce the risk of chronic illness
Digestive Function	Problems with digestion, such as constipation, diarrhea, or acid reflux; food sensitivities	Improved digestion and gut health
Respiratory Function	Difficult, rapid, or shallow breathing	Improved respiratory function, which can reduce risk of respiratory infections and optimize breathing efficiency

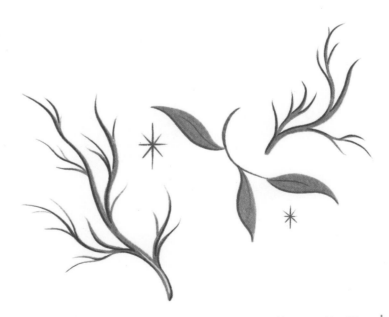

CAUSES OF LOW VAGAL TONE

Low vagal tone can be caused by a variety of factors, but some of the most common ones are outlined in this section.

Chronic Stress and Trauma

This is by far the most common contributor to low vagal tone. Prolonged exposure to stress or traumatic experiences can lead to an overactivation of the sympathetic nervous system, which can inhibit the vagus nerve. When you experience a threat (real or perceived), it changes your physiology. Usually you enter a fight-or-flight state, where your heart beats faster and you breathe more rapidly and shallowly— this is all a sympathetic nervous system response to help you fight or flee a threatening situation. Sometimes you may even enter a freeze or immobilized state, which again causes you to shallow breathe or even hold your breath. All of these states are facilitated by the vagus nerve. Something we see frequently in nature is that once safe, once the threat has passed, animals will release the stress response through shaking or breathing in some way to reset their baseline. Humans, however, will often stay in this chronic fight, flight, or freeze state for extended periods of time as a result of chronic stress or trauma. This unprocessed stress can lead to physical tension, restricted breathing patterns, posture issues, inefficient movement patterns, and high levels of stress hormones that can all negatively impact the functioning of the vagus nerve and further decrease resilience to stress over time.

Childhood Experiences

Adverse childhood experiences could include things like illness, injury, or even your mother's stress levels when you were in utero. There's research that shows that maternal stress, especially during the second trimester of pregnancy, may influence the physiological development of the baby's autonomic nervous system and lower vagal tone of the child. Again, this is not a life sentence. Vagal tone is not a rigid quality, so this is not an invitation for (A) any of you moms to reflect back on your pregnancy and feel any guilt for stress you experienced, or (B) any of you who know your mom was going through some hard things while pregnant to see it as unchangeable hardwiring. This is all just neutral information that might apply to your journey.

Chronic Inflammation

Chronic inflammation often refers to consistent, low-grade inflammation in the body and has been associated with low vagal tone. This reduction in vagal tone triggers the production of pro-inflammatory cells, which increase sympathetic nervous system activity and the release of stress hormones. Chronic inflammation can be caused by infections that don't go away, consistent consumption of inflammatory foods, stress, and autoimmune disorders—though it's important to keep in mind that the reason inflammation continues is not always known.

Medical Conditions or Physical Injury

There are many correlations between certain medical conditions and low vagal tone, but it's hard to tease out what caused what—did the medical condition decrease vagal tone or was low vagal tone a contributor to the condition? Findings suggest that diabetes, viral infections, abdominal surgeries, and scleroderma may be some of the conditions that can lead to some vagal nerve damage. Physical trauma or injury to the head, neck, spine, or chest may also damage the vagus nerve.

Lifestyle Factors

A variety of lifestyle factors have been associated with reducing vagal tone. Let's look at some of the most widely agreed-upon ones:

- **Sleep:** Sleep deprivation, or consistent low-quality sleep, is correlated with low vagal tone. Also, research shows that increasing vagal tone can significantly improve sleep quality.

- **Physical Activity:** Low levels of physical activity are correlated with low vagal tone, whereas an increase in physical activity can significantly improve vagal tone.

- **Nutrition:** The vagus nerve plays a huge role in our digestion, so it's no surprise that what we eat can impact vagal tone. High inflammatory foods like added sugar, hydrogenated oils, and refined carbohydrates can impair aspects of vagus nerve signaling, decreasing vagal tone.

- **Posture:** Poor posture can impact nerve blood flow and compress not only the vagus nerve but also various organs that the vagus nerve innervates, decreasing activity of the nerve.

- **Stress:** This bears mentioning again because I believe it's probably the leading cause of low vagal tone for most people. When we think about stress, it can help to examine different categories of stressors. Consider your environmental stress (clutter, heavy metals, mold, safety), relational stress, and work stress.

Substances and the Vagal Nerve

Here are some other substances that recent and ongoing research show may decrease vagal tone:

- Botox
- Antibiotics
- Alcohol
- Cannabis
- Heavy metals

Regardless of the cause, whether due to circumstances in utero, childhood trauma, or current life stressors, you are not stuck. Vagal tone is flexible and adaptable. Just as I said that regardless of your starting point there are specific things that can improve your muscle tone with intentional effort and consistency, the same goes for vagal tone. Regardless of your current vagal tone, or the reason for it, there are tangible, research-supported ways to improve it that will positively impact your overall well-being.

HOW TO ASSESS YOUR VAGAL TONE

Vagal tone isn't directly measured with a single test. Instead, it is measured with a variety of different tests all correlated with the various functions of the vagus nerve. The goal is to gain an overall picture of vagal function. Of all these tests, the one that is used most often and found to give the most accurate snapshot of vagal tone is heart rate variability (HRV), which we will soon cover in more depth. There are more formal tests you may have done in a physician's office, but I want to focus this section on things that you can do at home, including some things I have my clients do, to assess your vagal tone yourself. I split these assessments into three assessment categories: Symptom Clusters, Manual Assessments, and Device-Assisted Assessments.

Symptom Clusters

Remember that long list of symptoms in chapter 1, some of which likely resonated with you (see page 13)? Low vagal tone can be a common thread linking a series of seemingly unrelated symptoms. Symptoms of low vagal tone can vary depending on the underlying cause, but here are some common clusters associated with low vagal tone (and again, if you nod your head to more than one that's likely not a coincidence):

- Gastrointestinal issues like IBS, constipation, diarrhea, bloating, food intolerances, or acid reflux

- Low-quality sleep, insomnia (other sleep issues), fatigue, or headaches

- Chronic pain, aches, or muscle tension

- Autoimmune issues or other chronic conditions

- Sexual dysfunction

- Anxiety, emotional reactivity, or always feeling overwhelmed

- Depression, feeling disconnected, fatigue, lack of motivation

- Cardiovascular issues like high blood pressure or tachycardia

- Breathing issues like predominately mouth breathing, difficulty breathing, rapid breathing, or shallow breathing

Low vagal tone is likely not the singular cause of some of these—they may also be impacted by other psychological, endocrine, or relational factors—but your vagus nerve still has some role to play in each. It might feel like a game of "What comes first, the chicken or the egg?" Did your stress create short shallow breathing patterns that then negatively impacted vagal tone? Or did your low vagal tone impact your breathing in a way that added stress to your nervous system? Did low vagal tone impact your sexual dysfunction, which has created some relationship tension? Or did the relationship tension create sexual dysfunction and stress that may have impacted your vagal tone? I'm here to remind you to take a deep breath and not try to tease any of these things out because it might not matter. Almost all of these symptoms have a bidirectional relationship with vagal tone, meaning that improving vagal tone positively impacts symptoms. When you aim to decrease symptoms through other methods, that will likely positively improve your vagal tone as well.

Vagal tone refers to the efficiency of the vagus nerve's communication. Having low or poor tone impacts interoception and can cause a number of negative symptoms. Assessing symptom clusters can help clue in to your current vagal tone, bringing you one step closer to healing the vagus nerve and improving your mental and physical health.

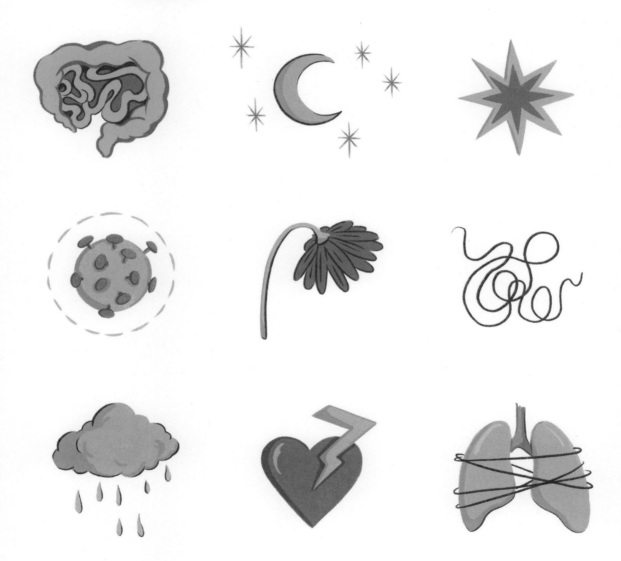

The bottom line is this: Improving your vagal tone will lead to overall improved mental and physical well-being, *and* making specific lifestyle, habit, and stress management shifts will positively impact your vagal tone. One step and one day at a time. Right now, we're not trying to improve anything yet; we're just trying to get a snapshot of your current vagal tone.

Manual Assessments

Manual assessments include observing your breathing patterns, doing a pharyngeal vagus branch test, and checking the transit time of food in the bowels.

Breath Observation

In chapter 2 we talked about what happens physiologically when we breathe. On the inhale, the lungs expand, the diaphragm flattens, and the heart rate speeds up. On the exhale, the lungs deflate, the diaphragm re-domes, and the heart rate slows down. A functional, optimal breath is an inhale through the nose, bringing the air down toward the belly, and exhaling out the nose. This full breath activates the vagus nerve, and each full breath is like one rep toward higher vagal tone.

Research shows that millions of adults breathe incorrectly, likely due to chronic stress and poor posture from sitting at a desk much of the day. So, observe your breath and see whether you have any of the following dysfunctions:

1. **Mouth breathing** (assess night and day)
   - When you mouth breathe, the vagus nerve is not properly stimulated, giving you less reps toward building high vagal tone. Mouth breathing is also a sympathetic stress signal to the nervous system.

   - To assess during the day, simply pay attention to how you breathe throughout the day and take note of how often you are nasal versus mouth

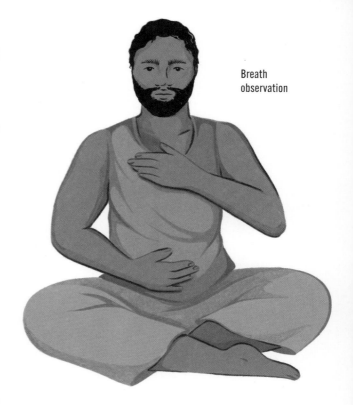

Breath observation

breathing. To assess during the night, some common signs that you might be sleeping with your mouth open include drooling, snoring, or having nasal obstructions. You could also consider asking a partner, if you have one, to note how you're breathing while sleeping.

2. **Shallow breathing**
   - To assess, observe your inhale. Does your chest or shoulders rise instead of your belly? If so, you're likely shallow breathing. You can also assess by lying on your back, on a hard surface, and putting your hands around your lower ribs. You should feel an effortless expansion of the lower ribs on the inhale and a slow collapse on the exhale. If your ribs remain motionless, your breath is too shallow (even if you belly moves with your breath).

3. **Rapid breathing**
   - To assess your respiration rate, sit down in a chair and try to relax. Count how many natural breaths you take in 1 minute and record the number. A normal respiration rate for an adult person at rest ranges from twelve to eighteen breaths per minute. If your number is higher than that, it indicates more rapid breathing.

4. **Difficulty breathing**
   - Breathing should be effortless, nonlabored, and have a regular rhythm. Take note of whether you experience any wheezing or difficulty breathing in any way.

Also note that there's a high correlation between posture and proper breathing, so if you know that you have poor posture, you also likely have some breathing dysfunction. These assessments will always be slightly objective because anytime you're paying attention to your breath it will likely deviate from its norm at least a little. Still, take note of any of these signs of dysfunctional breathing, because they could indicate low vagal tone.

Pharyngeal Vagus Branch Test

One of the branches of the ventral vagus nerve is called the pharyngeal branch. This test evaluates the movement of one of the muscles innervated by the pharyngeal branch, called the levator veli palatini muscle, which is the elevator muscle of the soft palate. The condition of this branch can be a good indicator of the function of other branches of the ventral vagus nerve as well.

To assess this one, you may need a partner. Here's how to do it:

- Grab a partner (or a mirror if no partner is available) and a flashlight.

- Look inside your mouth at the back of the throat where the uvula drops down in the center. You may want to use something to push down on your tongue so the uvula and soft palate above it are more visible.

- Make "ah, ah, ah" sounds.

- While making the sounds, your partner should look at the uvula to see whether there is any deviation to one side or the other or whether it goes symmetrically straight up as you make the sound.

If the uvula pulls over to one side, that is indicative of ventral vagal nerve dysfunction. If it moves up symmetrically, you are in a more regulated state, implying higher vagal tone. Overall improved vagal tone should allow it to rise more symmetrically.

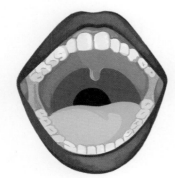

The uvula stays symmetrically straight up and down.

uvula

The uvula pulls over to one side.

Sesame Seed Bowel Transit Time

Sesame seeds come out looking the same as they went in, so we can use them to measure bowel motility by seeing how long it takes for a small amount of sesame seeds to pass through the digestive tract. All you need for this test is a teaspoon of sesame seeds, a cup of water, and a clock. So, if you're willing to give this a go, all you have to do is follow these four simple steps:

1. Mix a teaspoon of sesame seeds in a glass of room-temperature water.

2. Drink it all.

3. Write down the current time.

4. Wait and then observe.

It's probably obvious, but what you're watching for is a bowel movement containing the seeds. The ideal bowel transit time is anywhere from twelve to twenty-four hours. A transit time longer than two days means things are backed up in your digestive tract, increasing the risk of hormonal imbalances, diverticulosis, colon cancer, and candida. A transit time less than ten hours can mean a lack of nutrient absorption, leading to nutrient deficiencies or weakened immunity. Because the vagus nerve plays such a huge role in digestion, a deviation from ideal bowel transit time could indicate low functioning.

Device-Assisted Assessments

For these assessments, you will need a smart watch, fitness tracker, or device of some kind to track accurately. I've included these assessments because these devices are commonly worn and, in my opinion, worth the investment if you're serious about optimizing vagal tone—if for nothing else than to specifically track HRV, because it is currently the best way to measure vagal tone. Two other metrics I get from the device I use that are helpful are breath rate and sleep quality. See the Resources (page 148) for some of my current favorites to assist you in collecting this information.

Heart Rate Variability

As I previously mentioned, this test measures the variation in time (milliseconds) between your heartbeats, which is controlled by the vagus nerve. HRV gives a snapshot into how your body is balancing between the two branches of your autonomic nervous system—sympathetic activation and parasympathetic relaxation. High HRV is associated with higher vagal

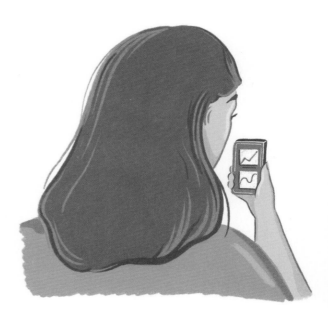

tone, more activation of your parasympathetic state, better resistance to stress, and overall physical well-being. Low HRV is associated with low vagal tone, more sympathetic activation, stress, illness, and more.

Many wearable devices will automatically track this throughout the day and especially during sleep. It is currently the most accurate and objective way to get a snapshot of your overall vagal tone and any changes to it over time.

Breath Rate

Breath rate measures how many breaths you take, on average, per minute. Most wearable devices will track this overnight as you sleep because that's when your body is in its most consistent state. This tracking uses something called respiratory sinus arrhythmia (RSA), which measures the changes in your heart rate that occur while breathing—when you breathe in, your heart rate increases; when you breathe out, your heart rate slows down. An average respiratory rate for healthy adults is twelve to eighteen breaths per minute. This is a helpful metric to track because it's very consistent. From night to night, your average breath rate should vary by only one or two breaths per minute. Any deviation greater than two breaths per minute is a sign worth paying attention to.

When my device tells me my breath or heart rate was higher than average on any given night, this usually means my body is under strain, typically from one of two things. Either I'm coming down with the latest bug my kid brought home from school or I'm carrying a higher stress load than normal and my body stayed in a more activated state throughout the night. This information helps me be mindful to build in intentional relaxation time the next day, say no to extra tasks, and be more compassionate toward myself when I notice I'm feeling extra annoyed or reactive.

Collecting data is only as helpful as how you decide to leverage that data to promote tangible behavior change. Knowing your average breath rate, or other measurements, can help you stay attuned to when a change occurs. Watching those patterns happen can give you some powerful real-time information on how to better support your well-being.

Sleep Quality

Sleep is one of the lifestyle factors that has the biggest ripple effect on your mental and physical well-being. When sleep quality diminishes, so does your mental and physical health. When sleep quality improves, so does just about everything else—and your overall vagal tone is no exception. Adequate sleep is crucial for the proper functioning of the vagus nerve, and I often see correlations between low vagal tone and low-quality sleep (and vice versa).

Most of the wearable devices use robust metrics throughout the night to assess sleep quality, usually tracking:

- **Total Sleep:** How much time you were asleep
- **Efficiency:** How long you were asleep relative to how long you were in bed
- **Latency:** How quickly you fell asleep
- **Sleep Cycle:** How much time you spent in each of the four sleep phases (awake, light sleep, REM sleep, deep sleep)
- **Timing:** When you're actually going to sleep and waking up (and whether that aligns with your body's natural circadian rhythm)

Again, the power in this information comes not just from tracking change over time but how you choose to leverage it on a day-to-day basis to motivate and inform helpful behavior change.

HOW TO CHOOSE YOUR METRICS

I just gave you a number of different ways to assess vagal tone. You absolutely do not need to do them all. You can do any, all, or none of the above (which means you just trust that doing some of the practices discussed in the next couple of chapters are going to support you!). When embarking on this journey to heal your vagus nerve, remember that stress plays a huge role. *Do not* stress yourself out thinking you need to assess and track everything in order to get a helpful snapshot—you do not. Some people are really motivated by metrics and tracking, and that's perfect. Others may not be, and that's perfect too. The following is a quick overview to help you decide which assessments might be the best fit for you.

Here's what I personally track, and what I typically have clients track:

1. **Symptom clusters:** I have clients track this through self-observation, conversations with me, and by filling out a symptom tracking survey each month.

1. **Breath observation:** Clients do this on their own and I will also do it in a session with them, tracking their starting point and any changes. For many of my clients, when we first start working together it feels hard or restrictive for them to take a deep breath, but with time and practice that gets easier. Sometimes they identify that they mouth breathe or shallow breathe. If so, I help them retrain optimal breathing practices and track changes.

2. **Device-assisted metrics**: These are my personal favorite ways to assess because it feels the easiest and most objective. It's definitely something I monitor for clients who have, or choose to get, a device. I look primarily at the data as outlined on pages 78 and 79.

If a client struggles specifically with digestive issues as a symptom cluster, they may also do the sesame seed bowel transit time assessment. What I track varies from client to client and often changes throughout our work together as certain metrics need more attention. I also have clients who feel overwhelmed by any kind of formal assessment tracking; that's okay too! If that's the case, we simply observe general trends and changes over time as they make supportive nervous system and lifestyle shifts.

It's essential to note that most of these metrics will be individual to *you*, meaning you should only compare changes relative to your own baseline and not with other people's data.

I invite you to take a quick look through this chapter again and choose one or two ways of assessing your vagal tone that feel helpful and not overwhelming. But whether you choose to formally assess your vagal tone or not, the suggestions made in the coming pages of this book are research-supported ways to activate your vagus nerve. When done consistently, they will improve vagal tone.

Once you have an idea of where you're starting, you're ready to take the next steps toward healing. The next chapter provides a framework for how to do that in a strategic and personalized way through a neuroscience- and trauma-informed lens.

QUICK SUMMARY

- Vagal tone is a measure of the activity and function of the vagus nerve.

- High vagal tone is a good thing and refers to a state in which the vagus nerve is active and functioning properly—sending signals to the body's organs and systems in a way that promotes balance and overall well-being.

- Low vagal tone refers to a state in which the vagus nerve is not active or functioning properly. It's not sending signals to the body in an effective or efficient way, which can contribute to a variety of symptoms and conditions.

- Chronic stress, trauma, medical conditions, and lifestyle factors can all contribute to low vagal tone.

- There are many ways to assess vagal tone. The clearest and most objective measure is heart rate variability (HRV). However you choose to assess, remember that measurements are unique to you. It's unhelpful to compare this data with other people's; simply track *your* changes over time.

5

HEALING THE VAGUS NERVE

Healing doesn't have to feel vague or ambiguous. A strategic and personalized framework for healing is key to regulating the nervous system.

The good news is that if you've already read the previous chapters, you've already begun healing your vagus nerve. The theory, the education, and the understanding of how this system works creates a new lens to use as you move through the world and your life. The context of how your system works gives you a deeper, and hopefully more compassionate, understanding of behavior and how these systems play a part in your everyday life. The thick educational and contextual foundation in the previous chapters is helpful to understand before trying to jump into any of the behavior changes. You see, urgency to heal is a sign you're still operating from survival mode, from dysregulation, and your nervous system isn't very flexible or willing to heal when it's in that place.

My hope is that by taking the time we did together to better understand your nervous system and the role of the vagus nerve, you've slowed down and made space for this work to happen at the pace that's right for *your* body. Improving vagal tone and regulating the nervous system takes time and repetition; if you're looking for overnight results you won't find them. I don't say this to be discouraging but to set you up for the very raw and real task of healing. It takes time and consistency, and I hope with all the context and knowledge you've gained up to this point you're feeling a healthy balance of groundedness, patience, and readiness to step into taking action to heal.

REMINDER: Higher vagal tone is associated with lower blood pressure, improved blood-sugar regulation, enhanced digestion, improved immune function, better mood, reduced anxiety, reduced risk of stroke and cardiovascular disease, improved ability to relax faster after stress, greater resistance to stress, better sleep, and better positive emotional responses. Cultivating higher vagal tone improves general nervous system function, increasing your ability to cope with daily life stressors without becoming overwhelmed and enhancing overall mental and physical well-being.

THE PROCESS OF HEALING

I once had a client come into session and share that the concept of "healing" felt overwhelming to her. She had questions like: What does *healing* even mean? What does it look like? Where do I start? How do I know whether it's working? And so on . . .

I laid out for her my four-phase neuroscience and trauma-informed formula of healing. I'd like to do the same for you to provide a framework and help answer those questions.

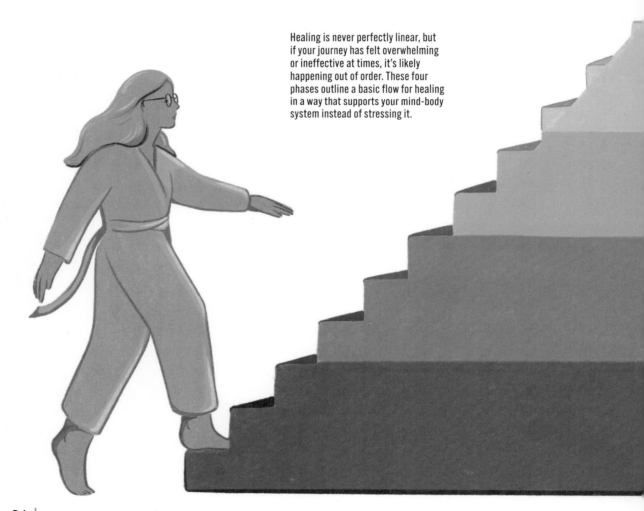

Healing is never perfectly linear, but if your journey has felt overwhelming or ineffective at times, it's likely happening out of order. These four phases outline a basic flow for healing in a way that supports your mind-body system instead of stressing it.

Phase 1: Education and Awareness

You've already explored this area with the previous chapters of this book. Understanding the nervous system theory as well as the science, and the role that your vagus nerve plays in it all, is fundamental and foundational to this work. If you don't understand how your system works, then you can't work with it toward healing. Then the awareness piece comes in anytime you personalize what you've learned to your unique experience of it with the nervous system mapping or symptom assessments.

Phase 2: Regulation

In this phase, you continue to learn the language of your nervous system. You get better at identifying when you're in dysregulation and start to implement reactive and proactive tools and practices that help you feel more grounded and regulated. With time and practice, you also start to identify the unique tools and strategies that work best for you in certain situations. This phase is rooted in some good old-fashioned trial and error to discover what works for you. Then you build on what works with consistent practice, collecting regulation reps over and over again, day after day. This is what we'll dive into shortly.

This is a crucial step before you dive into any deeper healing or repatterning work, what I refer to as the "rewiring phase." First you must prioritize building up the ability of your nervous system to regulate, and the capacity for your nervous system to move through discomfort, difficult emotions, and even trauma without becoming totally overwhelmed. In this phase, you learn how to regulate and to better understand the landscapes of each of your nervous system states, identifying the specific things that activate your system versus what helps you feel safe. If you don't do this work first, your system can get overwhelmed by attempts at cognitive reframing or trauma healing work, exacerbating symptoms.

Phase 4:
Resourcing

Phase 3:
Rewiring

Phase 2:
Regulation

Phase 1:
Education and Awareness

Phase 3: Rewiring

The first two phases form the foundation to create the capacity in your body for the deeper healing work to occur and to help you mitigate more stressors from coming in and getting trapped in your system. Once you have a more regulated baseline, as well as the necessary strategies to keep you connected and regulated, you now have the capacity to do some of the deeper work. This is where things like thought work, talk therapy, meditation, hypnotherapy, and parts work (ideally in combination with parallel somatic work) would come in. These are healing modalities that often work with the conscious mind to repattern thinking, behavior, and trauma responses. In my opinion, it can do more harm than good to dig into the vulnerable details that usually comes up in this work before first laying a proper foundation of regulation.

Phase 4: Resourcing

I often refer to this as "maintenance mode." This is where you continue to engage in the practices that are supportive for you, making small tweaks here or there depending on what you need to keep yourself at your new baseline. It's important to note that no one stays here forever. Inevitably, new triggers come up or life hands you a new situation outside your current ability to cope and you cycle back through these phases, but each time you do you'll notice you likely move through them with a little bit more ease and confidence from the previous healing work you've done.

This order and sequencing matters. When you jump too quickly into all the "vagus nerve stimulation practices" or "nervous system regulation hacks" without having an understanding of how those systems work and the unique role they play in anxiety, depression, chronic pain, or whatever you may be struggling with, you lack the context for how to integrate any of these practices intentionally. For example, a client shared that a few years prior she had a therapist who did a lot of the same things that she and I were doing in sessions—nervous system regulation work, somatic practices, breathwork, etc. But then she would go home and still be so dysregulated. She did not know how to do any of those practices on her own. What she came to realize during our work together was that no matter how helpful those practices were in a session, without the background education and awareness of how they impacted her system as a whole, she was totally dependent on another person to help her regulate.

Where I think most people go wrong is they try to jump right into rewiring with things like talk therapy, hypnotherapy, biohacking, or even psychedelics and plant medicines. All of these might do amazing things for some people or at a certain place in someone's healing journey. However, if your nervous system isn't ready for that big shift, then it can be ineffective at best or backfire in some serious ways at worst (by creating even more shutdown or fracturing). I'm not saying it does for everyone, but I can confidently say it does for many, many people, because I see it in my practice all the time. I've worked with countless individuals who've spent years in traditional talk therapy and their anxiety or depression isn't any better. In some cases, their symptoms have gotten worse. Without having the tools to stay present and regulated, your nervous system doesn't know the difference between the retelling of a traumatic experience versus actually re-experiencing it. Likewise with clients who tried a meditation or plant medicine retreat. Even a deep tissue massage can poke at the stored trauma in fascia and tissues, and make someone come out even deeper in a freeze response.

Here's the thing: Talking about your trauma or trying to access it through other channels is dysregulating. There's no way around that. If you don't have the capacity for additional dysregulation or know how to notice dysregulation happening in your system while having the ability to bring yourself back into a felt sense of safety and regulation, you're simply reinforcing the dysfunction and your need to stay in survival more. Before diving into deep rewiring work, you must first cultivate the capacity for it, and you do that through education, awareness, nervous system regulation, and vagal toning work.

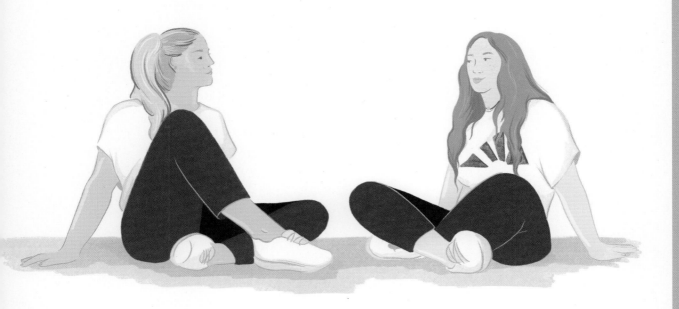

HEALING AND THE IMPORTANCE OF REPETITION OVER TIME

Improving vagal tone is a gradual process that requires regular practice and lifestyle changes. It's a balance of minimizing things that decrease vagal tone and increasing the practices and habits that activate the vagus nerve and improve vagal tone. In an attempt to simplify the often overwhelming concepts of "healing" or "nervous system regulation," here's another healing equation:

Improved Vagal Tone = Regulating Repetitions x Time

It's quite simple: The same way you improve muscle tone by accumulating repetitions of a weight-training exercise over time, improved vagal tone comes as the result of accumulating over time consistent reps of intentional practices and lifestyle changes that activate your vagus nerve and regulate your nervous system.

One of the most incredible things we've solidified in the last decade of research is that our nervous system is plastic, meaning it is forever changing and adapting in response to our thoughts, actions, and environment. If you can dysregulate your nervous system, you can regulate it too. We also know that the nervous system wants to heal; it wants to regulate. However, it can only do this when it's not prioritizing survival (stressors/environmental factors), and it does this through consistency and practice (reps x time).

Let's rewind for just a minute and talk about how the nervous system originally develops. When you are born, your autonomic nervous system (ANS) is only partially developed. At birth, the ANS is capable of controlling basic life-sustaining functions like regulating heart rate, breathing, and digestion. However, more complex functions like regulation of emotions and stress responses continue developing, and need support in properly developing, over the first few years of life and beyond. This maturing system is particularly vulnerable to adverse environmental, experiential, and social factors. Infants are *very* dependent on a human adult to co-regulate and connect. When a baby cries, a parent or caretaker swoops in to comfort or meet the needs of the infant, enabling them to come down out of their stress response. Day after day, over and over again, this baby learns that they're not alone and their needs will be met. As a child receives this co-regulation—has their needs met, feels loved and listened to, has boundaries set, is safe to express themselves, and all the things that tiny humans need—they develop an ability to self-regulate, which simply means they have the capacity to come out of a stress response on their own.

For the countless humans who didn't get that as a child, it's something they need to continue to learn as adults. Just like regulation would have been established day after day, rep after rep, influenced by the environment around a baby or child, healing your vagus nerve and rewiring your nervous system happens the same way as an adult.

What Slows Down Healing

Previously, I've mentioned the impact of how present stressors or your environment impact this work. Again, let's compare it to trying to improve muscle tone. You'll see a diminished rate of return on strength training if you're injured, poorly rested, or undereating—in fact, pushing too hard to build muscle under those conditions can impact you negatively. If your current environment or life situations are toxic and constantly dysregulating, you'll need to move slower through this work and consider starting with steps you can take to minimize stressors or create an environment more conducive to healing. The steps it'll take to do this will be unique to each individual, and seeking out professional support can be helpful.

Another thing that can slow down this healing work is trying to do too much too soon. I'll turn again to muscles to help explain. In weightlifting, if you lift too much too soon—before you have an understanding of how to do the exercise properly for your body and a baseline of strength and stability—you increase your chances of physical injury. Similarly, trying to change too much overnight increases stress load and reinforces your nervous system's need for survival mode. Ironically, the thing that speeds up this healing work the most is slowing down, decreasing the sense of urgency, and layering on regulating practices and lifestyle shifts little by little. The nervous system regulates and heals slowly, one regulating rep at a time.

MY HEALING JOURNEY

I remember my early healing journey feeling like a thousand-piece puzzle that I'd lost the box to. You know, the box with the picture on the front showing you what the finished puzzle looks like. Without that picture to go by, it felt like pieces were scattered everywhere and I didn't know where to start. I spent way too long feeling frustrated, stuck, and confused. For a while, I lived in denial of just how bad my anxiety was. I often chalked it up to "this is just how I am." Then the chronic overfunctioning eventually morphed into a depression I couldn't ignore anymore. I knew something had to change. I had to do something, but what?

I started with self-help, then eventually talked to my doctor, went to therapy, worked out, meditated, medicated, and more. I was trying anything and everything without ever quite feeling or healing in the way that I wanted to. It felt similar to throwing spaghetti at a wall just to see what stuck. I didn't just want to know why I was struggling; I wanted tangible tools to feel better. I didn't just want to take the edge off my symptoms; I wanted to get at the root of what was causing them. I craved a strategy. I needed a framework to help me organize my healing. Understanding the nervous system and the role of my vagus nerve allowed me to pump strategy into my healing in a really powerful and tangible way. Just like I had learned as a personal trainer and an athlete that there were strategic ways to strengthen and heal the body, I began to see that there were also research-supported and strategic ways to heal my mental health struggles. This framework is now the process I support clients in every day.

STRATEGIC HEALING

Before establishing my full-time mental health coaching practice, I spent almost a decade as a personal trainer and wellness specialist (hence all the strength-training analogies I use). I consistently and strategically created specific workout programs based on my clients' goals, current fitness level, and lifestyle. I took into consideration any limitations they had and the resources that were available to them. These plans were strategic but also flexible. Then things would be adapted and changed based on what we observed was working or not working for one reason or another as the client progressed. I apply this same process now to the anxiety and depression coaching that I do. Although there are many universals in how to improve both physical fitness and mental health, there is always a need for personalization and adaptation.

I believe in strategic healing and in creating an intentional plan of action to achieve your goals. I'm also a healing minimalist. My goal for clients, both when I was with them in the gym and now in my current mental health practice, has always been for them to get away with doing as little as possible to accomplish what they want. I support clients in finding the tools and practices that are the most effective for them and want to help you do the same. To do this, you will need to use the research-supported practices that universally support nervous system regulation and intimately observe how each of these practices uniquely impacts you.

The same way a comprehensive fitness program includes various categories of training, such as strength, cardio, core, flexibility, and stability, a strategic and comprehensive nervous system program also consists of various categories of training. To start, I've simplified this into two primary categories: proactive and reactive. Let's take a look at each.

PROACTIVE VERSUS REACTIVE HEALING TOOLS

In my coaching practice, we help clients create two very distinct toolboxes: one for proactive tools and the other for reactive tools. Too often in the support or messaging you get on a healing journey, there is overemphasis on one of these categories over the other. You need both.

Proactive practices include *consistent habits and lifestyle routines* to improve vagal tone and create a life more suited for nervous system regulation. These are things you do *proactively* to decrease the likelihood of dysregulation or your symptoms showing up. This includes things like sleep quality, movement, stress management, and vagal toning exercises. This category can eventually include the deeper cognitive and trauma healing work to lay down new patterns for your future as well. It is a response to statements like, "I want to be more regulated overall. I want a long-term game plan for healing."

Conversely, reactive practices are the *in-the-moment regulation exercises* that help you reverse the spiral of activation or shutdown. There are countless ways to do this, but these tools typically focus on helping you come back into connection with your body and environment in the present moment through your senses or specific practices that activate the vagus nerve. This toolbox is in response to statements like "I'm already there. I'm activated, I'm triggered. Or even I'm shut down. Now what?"

Proactive Healing Tools

When it comes to proactive healing, there are nine research-supported categories that contribute to overall improved regulation and vagal tone that I use as guidelines in my coaching practice. Here they are with brief descriptions and some research-supported guidelines I often make for clients in each of these categories (always filtering it through their unique needs, their capacity, and the resources available to them).

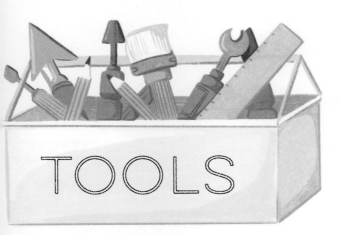

Proactive Habit	Overview and Guidelines
1 **Sleep**	Sleep is the most fundamental player in our mental and physical health, and the vagus nerve plays an important role in the regulation of sleep. Set a goal to make sure that you sleep long enough and deep enough 80 percent of the nights of your life. Research often categorizes quality sleep as an average of eight hours a night, with consistent timing (when you go to bed and wake up each day). Ideally, you're able to wake up without an alarm feeling rested.
2 **Movement**	Movement and exercise have a positive impact on the vagus nerve, and research makes it clear that the healthiest version of your brain lives within a body in motion. There's a lot of nuance and personalization when it comes to a movement routine, but some general guidelines are to aim for 150+ minutes of heart-pumping physical activity per week, but even a short daily walk can make a difference.
3 **Breath**	Breathing is a key way you can influence the vagus nerve. Slow, deep breathing stimulates activity of the vagus nerve, promoting relaxation and reducing the stress response. Breath has a powerful proactive and reactive impact on our well-being. You want to take proactive steps toward a functional breathing pattern, which looks like diaphragmatic breathing in and out through your nose.
4 **Vagal Toning Practices**	Just like there are specific exercises to activate your biceps or abs, these are specific exercises or practices used to activate the vagus nerve. These can be used reactively in the moment to regulate or proactively to improve vagal tone. The next chapter includes examples of and instructions for many vagal toning practices, beginning on page 104.
5 **Gut Health**	The gut and vagus nerve are closely interconnected, which means poor gut health can lead to inflammation and immune dysfunction that negatively impact the activity of the vagus nerve. Some general gut-healthy guidelines are to eat a diverse and healthy diet of whole foods; take probiotics and/or eat fermented foods; manage stress; improve sleep; avoid taking antibiotics when possible; and minimize or eliminate added sugars, vegetable oils, and trans fats because they all cause inflammation in the gut. Improving gut health can be a very individualized process and it is often worth talking to a gut specialist.

Proactive Habit	Overview and Guidelines

 Vision Therapy

The visual system is a strong lever you can pull to shift the state of your mind and body. Vision is the dominant sense that humans use to navigate the world and survive, and there are very interesting interactions between how you see and how you feel internally. Stress changes your vision, and by intentionally shifting your vision you can decrease (or increase) the stress response. Stress activates a type of tunnel vision. Convergence, meaning your eyes moving together to look at something close up (like your phone), activates the sympathetic nervous system. Engaging in distance viewing, scanning, or intentionally focusing on your peripheral vision decreases the body's stress response. Overall, vision therapy is designed to improve visual function and enhance the connection between the eyes and the brain. There's limited research on the specific impacts of vision therapy on the vagus nerve, but some evidence suggests it has a positive impact on vagal activity through its effects on stress and relaxation. The following chapter provides vision therapy drills, beginning on page 112. My experience has shown that balancing time spent looking close up at screens versus distance viewing out a window or while on a walk generally has positive overall effects as well.

 Community

The parasympathetic state can activate and be activated through social connection. Research has found that high-quality social interactions can protect against trauma, depression, and other mental health issues. That's because healthy social connection engages the parasympathetic response and activates your vagus nerve. When the vagus nerve has high tone, it better equips you to respond, listen, and engage with others. Do you currently feel like you have quality social interactions? Are you able to set boundaries on relationships or interactions that feel draining or dysregulating? Identifying and spending time with people who make you feel safe and supported is the goal. Intentionally cultivating this will positively impact vagal tone.

 Repatterning: Mindset and Trauma Healing

Trauma leads to dysregulation of the autonomic nervous system, decreased vagal activity, and protective thinking patterns. By repatterning protective/problematic thinking and releasing stored trauma in the body, you can reduce hypervigilance and stress while improving emotional regulation and immune function. Working with a trauma-trained professional is often the best route to take for this work.

 Environment and Stress Management

Research makes it clear that each person's environment and stressors significantly impact their nervous system state. Environment can include things like air or noise pollution, clutter, and toxic social environments that increase the body's stress response. Managing your overall stress load and being mindful of creating or spending time in less stressful environments will positively impact vagal tone.

Remember, the goal isn't to overhaul your life overnight; in fact, I strongly recommend that you focus on one, *maybe* two, of these habits at a time. Also, know that a lot of times you may need support in establishing sustainable behavior change (this is a huge part of the work I do with clients).

A good place to start is to decide which of these categories feels the easiest to shift, or which one has the biggest impact for you, and start there. Make a small shift in a helpful direction, repeat that long enough that it becomes your new baseline habit, and then either make another small shift in that same area or move to a new habit to shift in a small way. The goal is to start small, collecting reps of the improved habit until it becomes your new baseline.

Here are some guiding questions on how you can figure out where to start:

- Which of these habits makes the biggest difference for me? I often ask clients, "What's your number one proactive self-care practice? Which one of these things, when it happens consistently and with high quality, makes the biggest difference in how you feel overall? Which one of these, when done consistently makes it hard for you to have your *worst* day?"

- Let's say for you it's sleep. Now ask yourself, what do my current habits around sleep look like? What's stopping me from getting enough quality sleep? What is one, small step I could take toward improving this?

- Let's say you notice you scroll on your phone for a while before bed. Maybe you start by plugging in your phone on your dresser instead of your nightstand; that way, you aren't bringing it to bed with you. Maybe you set an alarm ten minutes before you'd like to go to bed as a reminder to put your phone away and go brush your teeth.

If ten minutes feels too hard, start with five. If an alarm isn't working, then maybe choose a time in the day to delete the apps that are the most tempting for you. The goal with behavior change is to start small and have obvious cues for your new behavior. You want to make it as easy as possible to do the things you want to do (get off your phone earlier) and add barriers that make it harder to do things you don't want to do (scrolling late into the night).

When coaching clients, I help them walk back their behavior change until it feels almost laughably small. For example, a client was struggling with morning anxiety and wanted to have a morning routine (she currently had none). They had set the goal to wake up thirty minutes earlier to meditate and go for a walk before getting ready for work, but they'd set that goal over a month before and had only made it happen once. Setting a goal to go from no morning routine to a thirty-minute multistep morning process sounds nice, but it also sets you up for failure.

Here's how the next part of that conversation went:

Me: "What's the tiniest step you can take toward this ideal morning routine?"

Client: "I could just do the ten-minute meditation."

Me: "Even tinier."

Client: "Maybe I'll do just a five-minute meditation."

Me: "Could you make that even tinier?"

Client: "Anything shorter than that feels like it doesn't even matter."

Me: "What difference might taking just three deep breaths when you first wake up make?"

Client: "I guess it would be something, more than I'm doing right now."

Me: "Exactly. And how confident do you feel that tomorrow morning before getting out of bed you could take three deep breaths?"

Client: "That feels easy; I'm totally confident I could do that."

Me: "Great, let's start there."

BINGO.

Here's the reality: This client had decided multiple times in the past few months to establish a more intentional mindful morning routine but every time they only kept up the habit for a day or two. After two weeks of "all I have to do is take three deep breaths, anything else is a bonus," they kept steadily layering on to their morning routine. They eventually made it to where most days they automatically wake up and slip right into an intentional and regulating ten- to twenty-minute (they realized they didn't even need the full thirty minutes to create regulation) morning routine that curbs their anxiety and starts their day off at a much better place. To proactively shift in a more

helpful and regulating direction, you must first install a tiny habit and then optimize it from there.

I'll say it again: You must start laughable small. You need to choose a version of that new desired behavior that, even on your worst days, when you feel like doing nothing, you can think, "Well, it's only three breaths" or "All I have to do is take three breaths, nothing more if I don't want to."

When it comes to changing habits, it's hard. In my practice, I often hear phrases like, "I know what I should be doing to feel better, but I can't get myself to do it." Then they assume it's because of lack of motivation or willpower. Well, I just don't believe that. You do what you have the capacity to do, and you're hardwired to keep doing what you've been doing, especially when you're stressed out. The truth is that positive life changes lead to positive brain changes, and those positive brain changes support you in making more positive life changes. (See the Resources section, page 148, for a couple of other books I love on creating habits.)

Regulating your nervous system and healing your vagus nerve means changing the way you live your life in at least some way. And, as I've previously noted, making those changes can be hard and frequently requires support and additional capacity. What often helps create the capacity to make some of the grander life changes is being able to push back on your body's stress response in real time. I help clients do this by identifying the reactive, in-the-moment coping tools that help them feel more regulated and in control.

Reactive Healing Tools

Reactive healing tools provide in-the-moment support to help you push back against the body's stress response in real time to activate your vagus nerve and regulate your nervous system. After my clients gain an awareness of their nervous system and can identify which state they are experiencing in any given moment, identifying a few reactive regulating practices is one of the very next things we do—even before trying to proactively change any habits. Learning how to notice dysregulation occurring in the moment and having tools you're confident will support you in feeling more grounded immediately is incredibly empowering. You'll also find that accumulating these regulation reps creates more capacity for the other healing work.

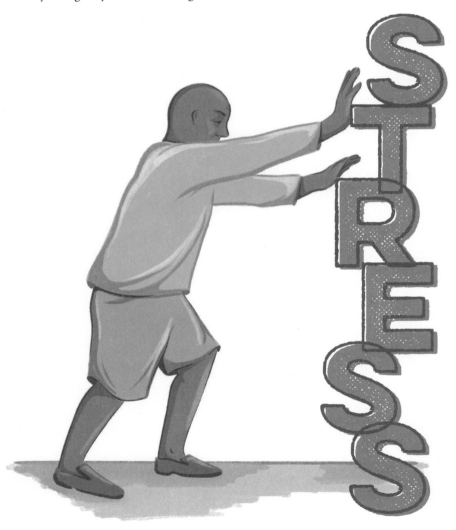

Here are a few things to remember when it comes to creating your reactive healing toolbox:

- Some tools or practices may be universally regulating for you, while others are beneficial depending on which nervous system state you are in. Don't skip over the awareness phase of learning to identify when you're in states of activation versus shutdown, as that awareness will inform which reactive tools you'll want to turn to first.

- Consistency is key! Bringing regulation to your nervous system requires consistent neural exercises (e.g., things that move your system toward regulation). Again, just like doing reps at the gym, muscle reps over time = muscle toning. Regulating reps over time = vagal toning.

- Reactive tools should also be practiced proactively. If you only use these regulating resources when you are in distress, it will be challenging to use them because you haven't practiced. Without consistent practice, you won't be reshaping your nervous system. The key is to identify specific tools or practices you already engage in that help you feel more regulated.

- Plan to sprinkle in reactive tools throughout your day. For some people that might be three times a day; for others that could be ten times a day. It should feel intentional but not overwhelming.

- The goal when regulating isn't to jump right into the green zone, feeling perfectly calm and grounded. The goal is to move even just one tiny step toward regulation. If you go from level 8 sympathetic activation to a level 7, that's great! More regulation can come from repeating the practice or layering on others.

- Identifying which regulation practices are the best fit for you takes some intentional exploration and some good old-fashioned trial and error.

When reactively regulating, you first need to meet your system where it is (activation or shutdown) and then slowly move it toward regulation.

Reactive Regulation When in Activation

You're feeling anxious and you know this means you're in a state of sympathetic activation. You might think, "Okay, the goal is to calm down, so I'm going to take a deep breath or try a meditation to bring in more stillness." But remember, being in this state changes your physiology to promote mobilization, so jumping right into stillness might actually activate your nervous system even more rather than help it. This is why so often people write off things like meditation or breathwork as something that "doesn't work for them" when the reality might be that they were just using it at the wrong time. Instead, you often need to meet your nervous system *in motion* first to allow that activated energy to discharge and leave your body. This could look like giving your body a quick shake, going for a walk, or even clenching and opening your fists. You'll know a practice is supportive if you start to feel more settled and less urgent, are able to release tension, or can breathe more deeply—even if that shift is subtle. Think about this like the "up" state and the goal is to down-regulate one step at a time.

Reactive Regulation When in Shutdown

You're feeling depressed, maybe even a bit disconnected or dissociated—you know this means you're in a state of dorsal vagal shutdown. The thoughts you often think here sound like, "I can't do anything" or "It doesn't matter." But for a moment, imagine with all the new context you have, you think instead, "Okay, the goal is to get into motion in some way, so I'm going to try to work out." Again, remember, being in this state changes your physiology to promote immobilization, so yes, an activated workout could be helpful to shift gears, but it's likely too much too fast. This is why the generic advice of "exercise is good for depression" can be so unhelpful because (A) you likely don't have the capacity to go from feeling so low to jumping into a bootcamp class, and (B) it might be too much too soon for your system even if you could willpower your way there (which I don't recommend). When in this red zone state, you aren't looking to come directly into that ventral vagal regulated state, as great as that would be. You're instead looking for small amounts of mobilizing energy to come into your body to feel just a bit more "here" or connected. Think about it like a bear slowly coming out of hibernation. This could look like moving from your couch to the porch, rubbing your hands together to bring awareness back to your body, or walking to the kitchen to drink a glass of cold water. You'll know a practice is supportive if you start to feel more in your body, aware of your surroundings, more capable and able, or a bit more energetic. Think about this like the "down" state and the goal is to up-regulate one step at a time.

You are able to heal the vagus nerve and reshape your nervous system through seemingly small steps. Every time you use a proactive or reactive regulating resource, you show your system that you're a little bit safer than it thought. You activate your vagus nerve and tap into your parasympathetic state. Doing this consistently improves vagal tone and creates a more regulated nervous system.

The next chapter will provide a wealth of guided practices you can start to explore and experiment with.

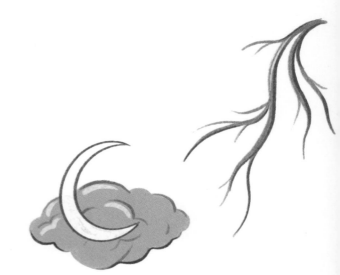

QUICK SUMMARY

- Healing = Regulating reps x time

- Improving vagal tone is a gradual process that requires regular practice and lifestyle changes.

- It is possible, and in my opinion essential, to engage in strategic healing. This comes from understanding how the vagus nerve operates and how to work with that physiology to regulate and move toward healing.

- Proactive regulation practices include sleep, movement, breath, vagal toning practices, gut health, vision therapy, community engagement, repatterning, and environmental and stress management. They also include proactively using reactive regulation practices you've identified as helpful for you to familiarize your system with them and make them more accessible practices in times of high stress.

- Reactive regulation practices are the in-the-moment tools that help you shift from a state of dysregulation toward regulation. In this you must first meet your nervous system where it is and slowly layer on tools or practices that move you toward regulation.

6

SOMATIC AND VAGAL TONING EXERCISES

Strong vagal tone is built the same way as strong muscles. Seemingly small but consistent repetitions over time make all the difference.

As you read this chapter, remember there's no one magic tool or trick; rather, there are countless different somatic and vagal toning practices that, when used consistently over days, months, and even years, can provide immense amounts of healing. Through some experimentation, you'll learn which tools are the best fit for you. This chapter is designed to be a library of guided practices to refer back to again and again.

In this chapter, you'll find a mix of both somatic and vagal toning practices. Both are aimed at regulating the nervous system and, in doing so, contributing to improved vagal tone. I want to take a moment to point out the difference between these categories of practices so if you hear these terms used elsewhere, you have more context. Somatic practices encompass a broader range of techniques aimed at addressing the mind-body connection, releasing physical tension, and healing trauma. Vagal toning exercises specifically target the vagus nerve to activate the body's relaxation response and promote overall well-being.

These tools are also a mix of proactive and reactive tools (page 91). Many of them can be used either way: as tools to proactively improve vagal tone, or reactively as in-the-moment practices to reverse the spiral of activation or shutdown. Keep in mind that even reactive tools should not be used exclusively for moments of distress. They need to be practiced proactively and in smaller moments of stress so that they become familiar and natural practices to use in the bigger moments of dysregulation.

On the following pages, you'll find a how-to guide for various practices. I've grouped them into three categories: vagal toning exercises, tools for activation, and tools for shutdown.

PREPARING FOR PRACTICE

Before trying some of these practices, I want to give you a framework for assessing the effectiveness of each for you. The goal is not to pursue all these practices, but instead to identify the ones that have the biggest payoff for you.

With many of the basic lifestyle and vagal toning practices such as exercise, gargling, and sunlight, the goal is to *proactively* build these practices into your daily life in a consistent and sustainable way. Just like most everyone's muscles break down and build back up in the same way with weight training, these practices seem to improve vagal tone somewhat universally for everyone—though of course everyone makes their gains at a different rate. The means for assessing is simply watching for increased capacity and change over time.

When it comes to using practices *reactively* for states of fight, flight, freeze, or shutdown, there's a simple way to tune in, check in, and assess effectiveness. Remember, different tools work for different states and different tools work more or less effectively for different people depending on the unique needs of their nervous system. When trying new practices, follow these steps:

1. **Choose a Baseline Assessment:** Tune in and identify which state you're in and the intensity of those sensations. I've included a guided baseline assessment as the first practice in this chapter. In addition to that subjective guided mind-body assessment, I often have clients do a more objective assessment observing a range of motion or physical tension in their body with stretches. What they often find, if a tool was helpful in creating more regulation, is that when retesting the same stretch they have less muscle tension and greater range of motion. Some of the most commonly used stretches are neck turns/tilts and a standing toe reach. A baseline assessment is simply tuning in—this can be done as an internal state assessment and/or a physical tension assessment.

2. **Insert a Regulating Practice:** Choose a practice and do it. Note that changing *how* you do a particular practice can also yield different results. Many practices have some flexibility to adjust frequency, duration, or intensity.

3. **Reassess:** Repeat the same baseline state assessment and/or body tension assessment and note any changes.

If you're activated, insert a tool, and then feel more settled or calm—even a tiny bit—it worked. Or, if you're shut down, insert a tool, and then feel more connected or energized—even a tiny bit—it worked.

If with any practice you notice decreased tension or an increased range of motion (in other words, there's decreased tension when you turn your head to the right or you're able to get closer to reaching your toes), then the practice was supportive in bringing your system more ease.

Other indicators a practice is working to reset your nervous system is if during or just after you yawn or sigh, notice deeper breathing, feel sensations of your GI tract coming back online (i.e., gurgling stomach, passing gas, burping), or simply feel more settled and present. Those are all signs that your vagus nerve has been activated and that the tool you just tried was supportive.

Some of the practices you'll find in this chapter are specific to activating your vagus nerve, while others are more general somatic and nervous system regulation practices. Anytime we move our nervous system toward regulation we are improving vagal tone.

BASELINE ASSESSMENT

This is a practice to help you engage interoception and collect a baseline for the current state of your nervous system. When experimenting with new regulation practices, it's important to do a brief check-in before using the tool so you have a baseline to help you better assess the effectiveness of that tool. This in-the-moment check-in will eventually become quicker and more automatic, but like most things we've never done before, we have to start intentionally and with some guidance.

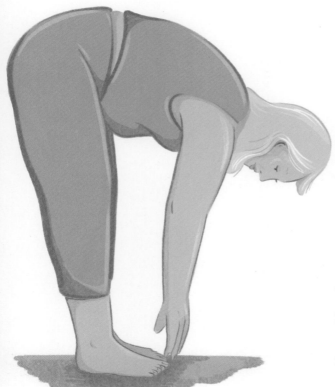

For this assessment, you'll first do a quick objective mobility assessment and then take a moment for your subjective baseline assessment where you will try to identify the current state of your mind and body. Then you'll give yourself a score on a scale of 1 to 10.

- **Mobility Assessment:** Turn or tilt your head right to left, or do a standing forward fold (where you reach for your toes). As you do this stretch or movement, notice any limitation in range of motion or muscle tension. You might also note if it feels different on one side of your body than the other.

- **State Assessment:** Take a moment to notice the qualities of your mind and sensations in your body. Do they align more with being shut down, activated, or regulated? You may also want to score it on a scale of 1 to 10 (just how regulated, activated, or shut down do you feel). Which zone/state does it feel like in your mind? What zone/state does it feel like in your body?

1. Red Zone = shut down, numb, disconnected, flat

2. Yellow Zone = activated, busy, thoughts or heart racing, hard time sitting still

3. Green Zone = regulated, present, calm

REMEMBER:

There's no right or wrong, or good or bad score. You're simply tuning in to see where you are so that you can measure any changes that occur as a result of the regulating practice you try.

1. Take a moment to pause what you're doing to tune in to your mind and body. If it feels safe and helpful for you, try closing your eyes.

2. Now bring your awareness to your mind. What is it like to be in your mind right now? Are your thoughts racing, jumping from one thing to the next? Is it hard to stay focused? If so, you're likely in the yellow zone. If your thoughts are present and attentive, assign yourself as being mentally in the green zone. If your thoughts feel distant, numb, or flat, note that you're in the red zone.

3. Now shift your awareness into your body. What is it like to be in your body right now? Do you feel antsy or agitated? Maybe you feel your heart racing or it's hard to sit still? If so, you're likely in the yellow zone. If you feel connected, energized but grounded, and present in your body, then you're more aligned with the green zone. If you're having a hard time connecting to or even feeling your body, or maybe it feels numb or flat, you're likely in the red zone.

4. Keep this in mind and repeat this awareness exercise (along with a mobility assessment if you choose to do that) after engaging in a regulating practice to see whether you notice any change in how you feel. Remember, some shifts can feel subtle, so the more often you tune in, the more aware you will become of those small shifts.

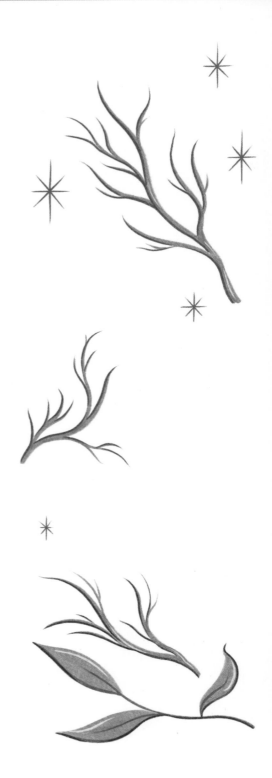

VAGAL TONING EXERCISES

The exercises and techniques in this section stimulate the vagus nerve and improve vagal tone. These are most effective at improving vagal tone when built into your daily life consistently, but they can also be used as reactive tools when you're in moments of dysregulation to help engage your parasympathetic state.

Remember to note any of these practices that bring on a sigh, swallow, yawn, turning on of the digestive track, or general settling in your body; these can all be signs of vagus nerve activation. Take note of any other changes in body sensations, breathing, and body tension.

These vagal toning practices are organized into five categories:

1. Breathing Exercises
2. Massage Techniques
3. Vision Exercises
4. Other Practices
5. Practitioner- and Device-Supported Techniques

Breathing Exercises

Consciously breathing in a certain way is one of the quickest levers you can pull to shift the state of your mind and body. These practices can be done as formal breathwork sessions where you set aside time, typically 5 to 10 minutes, to intentionally practice one of these techniques. You can also integrate each of these breath practices throughout your day for a simple series of three breaths, for 1 minute, or however you see fit. Instructions are written as if you're doing it in a more formal breath practice, but know that you can do most of these while sitting at your desk, watching a show, or doing just about anything else as a way to promote and practice functional breathing patterns that improve vagal tone.

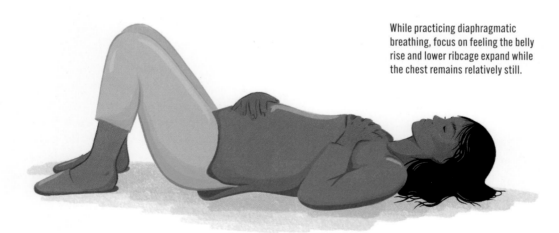

While practicing diaphragmatic breathing, focus on feeling the belly rise and lower ribcage expand while the chest remains relatively still.

Diaphragmatic Breathing

Diaphragmatic breathing is also sometimes referred to as belly breathing. This is how babies naturally breathe, yet most people develop dysregulated breathing patterns by adulthood—meaning things like shallow chest breathing or mouth breathing. By taking deep, slow, diaphragmatic breaths you activate the vagus nerve. By practicing this intentionally, the hope is that this breathing pattern becomes your normal and natural way of breathing throughout the day.

1. Find a comfortable, quiet place to sit or lie down.

2. Close your eyes (optional) and focus on your breath.

3. Place one hand on your chest and the other on your belly, somewhere below your ribs but above your belly button.

4. Take a slow, deep inhale through your nose, inviting the breath downward so that your belly rises underneath your lower hand. Your chest should remain relatively still, and your shoulders should not lift as you inhale. You should also feel your lower ribs expanding in your front, side, and back body.

5. Exhale slowly through your nose, allowing your belly to fall back down toward the spine. If you're having a hard time controlling the rate of your exhale, you can try exhaling out of your mouth while imagining you are slowly breathing out through a straw.

6. Repeat this pattern, bringing the inhale back in slowly through your nose, followed by an equal-length exhale. Focus on the sensation of your breath moving in and out of your body for 5 to 10 minutes.

Extended Exhale Breath

With this breath practice the focus is on extending your exhale out longer than your inhale. An extended exhale helps promote activation of the parasympathetic nervous system, calming and relaxing the body.

1. Find a comfortable, quiet place to sit or lie down.

2. Close your eyes (optional) and focus on your breath.

3. Inhale slowly and deeply through your nose for a count of 4.

4. Exhale slowly and fully through your nose or mouth for a count of 6.

5. Repeat this pattern for several minutes or until you feel a settling within your body.

The specific timing of the inhale and exhale counts can vary depending on individual needs and preferences. You can also experiment with adding a 2- or 3-second breath hold at the top of the inhale and bottom of the exhale. The most important thing is to find a rhythm that feels comfortable and natural for you.

Physiological Sigh

A physiological sigh is a breath pattern done naturally when trying to fall asleep or resetting after something stressful or a good cry. It's especially obvious as children start to wind down from being upset. You can also engage this breath pattern intentionally anytime you're feeling stressed and want to feel calmer. A physiological sigh is a pattern of breathing that involves two inhales followed by an extended exhale. You do it with two inhales, and typically the first inhale is longer than the second, followed by an extended exhale out through the mouth.

1. For this practice don't worry about finding any formal setting. Wherever you are is fine and closing your eyes is totally optional.

2. Take two inhales through your nose. A deep first inhale, immediately followed by another inhale.

3. Then give one long exhale through the mouth.

4. Repeating this breath just one to three times is sufficient to bring your level of stress down.

"Voo" Breath

This breath involves making a low-pitched humming sound during the exhale that activates the vagus nerve and promotes relaxation, stress reduction, and improved breathing function.

1. Find a comfortable, quiet place to sit or lie down.

2. Close your eyes and take a few deep breaths to relax your body.

3. On your next exhale, begin to make a low-pitched humming "voo" sound, similar to the sound of a bee or motorboat.

4. Allow the sound to vibrate through your body and focus on the sensation as you exhale.

5. Continue to make the humming sound for several exhales, or as long as you feel comfortable.

6. When you're ready, take a few more natural deep breaths and then slowly open your eyes.

Valsalva Technique

This breathing technique involves holding your breath while bearing down. You may have instinctively done this before to equalize pressure in your ears while swimming or flying. The vagus nerve plays a key part in the reflex triggered by this technique. It's important to note that this breathing technique can cause a sudden increase in blood pressure and is not recommended for everyone.

1. Sit or stand in a comfortable position.

2. Take a deep breath in through your nose.

3. Pinch your nose closed, close your mouth, and hold your breath.

4. Bear down as if you are trying to have a bowel movement, while keeping your mouth and nose closed.

5. Hold this position for 10 to 15 seconds, or until you feel a pressure sensation in your ears.

6. Open your mouth, unpinch your nose, and slowly release the breath.

7. Wait at least a minute before repeating; repeating this more than three times is not recommended.

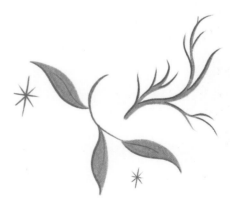

Massage Techniques

Vagus nerve massages don't directly massage the vagus nerve but rather areas that are in close enough proximity to the vagus nerve to provide some amount of stimulation and activation. Long-term improvements of heart rate variability have been seen with regular vagus nerve work through massage. Here you'll find instruction on how and where to massage your body to stimulate your vagus nerve.

Ear Massage

The nerve endings in your ear send afferent signals back to your brain, meaning if you stimulate the vagus nerve through your ear it sends a direct signal of calm back to your brain. This auricular branch of the vagus nerve also connects to facial nerves, so this can promote facial relaxation as well. When massaging the ear, focus on moving the skin versus applying pressure, you don't actually need much pressure at all here. There shouldn't be any pain or discomfort with these practices. Here are a few ways to massage the ear for vagus nerve stimulation.

Behind Ear Massage

1. Place your index finger behind the bottom back of your ear, behind your earlobe. Your fingertip will land in the valley behind your ear where it attaches to your skull.

2. Massage from bottom to top around the curve of your ear where it attaches to your head.

3. Repeat on the other side.

Concha Massage

1. Place your index finger in the little hollow just above and outside your ear canal.

2. Make gentle circles, or a back-and-forth movement, focusing on sliding the skin around.

3. Repeat on the other side.

Gentle Ear Pull

1. Very gently pull on your earlobe and hold for a period of time. This is also considered a craniosacral technique and can have benefits for dizziness, headaches, and other neurological-type symptoms.

Behind the Ear

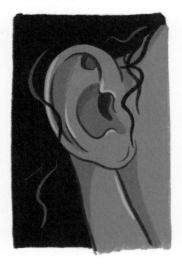

Concha Message

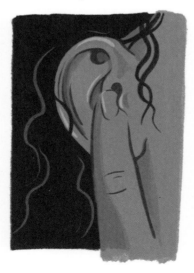

Gentle Ear Pull

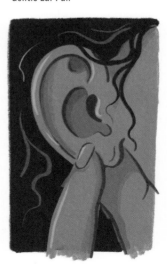

Neck Massage

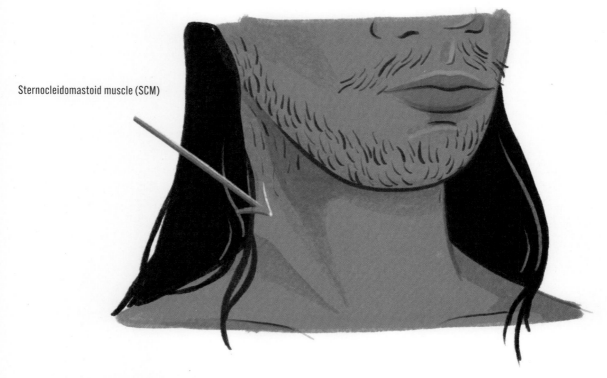

Sternocleidomastoid muscle (SCM)

Massaging most parts of your neck puts you in close enough proximity to stimulate the vagus nerve, but two primary areas to focus on are the sternocleidomastoid muscle (SCM) and the carotid sinus. The sternocleidomastoid is the muscle that runs along the side of your neck on both sides. When you turn your head to the side, you'll see a muscle pop out running from behind your ear down toward your clavicle—this is the SCM. The carotid sinus, which the vagus nerve innervates, is located just below the curve of your jaw and just inside the SCM. Massaging relaxes this muscle, and others commonly involved in stress breathing, and the pressure of the massage presses into the carotid sinus area. In activating the vagus nerve, this type of massage can bring down heart rate, lower breath rate, and induce a relaxation response.

I often combine my ear massages with a neck massage on each side and this is something that I love to do daily, but more realistically end up doing consistently three or four times a week.

Instruction for sternocleidomastoid muscle (SCM) massage

1. Find the SCM muscle. To do this, place your fingers on the side of your neck, just below your earlobe, and slowly turn your head to the opposite side. You should feel a long, thin muscle under your fingers. This is the SCM muscle.

2. There are a few ways to massage this muscle. You can apply gentle to moderate pressure and move in either an up or a downward motion. You can apply pressure with your fingers and move them in a circular motion. You can apply gently squeezes of this muscle between your thumb and index finger as you move up or down the muscle from behind your ear to the clavicle. You can also rub along this muscle.

3. You may also choose to pause and massage at the base of the SCM where it meets with the trapezius.

4. Work slowly, taking your time with the massage. Avoid applying too much pressure and instead focus on applying a steady, moderate pressure that feels comfortable and soothing.

5. Repeat on the other side.

Instructions for carotid sinus massage

NOTE: Massaging the carotid sinus to stimulate the vagus nerve can be dangerous if not done correctly because of its proximity to your carotid artery. Manipulating the carotid sinus incorrectly can result in a drop in blood pressure or heart rate. If you think you'd benefit from vagus nerve stimulation in this way, consult with a qualified health care professional who can guide you through how to appropriately and safely follow the steps below.

1. The vagus nerve runs up the neck just lateral to the carotid artery. Place your hand on the side of your neck until you can feel your carotid pulse, then move just behind and lateral to that and you'll feel some tissue.

2. With two or three fingers, gently make small circles, moving your way up and down the side of your neck. Remember, the key here is to be extremely gentle; pushing too hard on the carotid artery can have negative effects.

3. Repeat on the other side.

Abdominal Massage

The vagus nerve runs through the abdomen, so perhaps it's no surprise that stimulating this area through abdominal massage can promote stimulation of the vagus nerve as well as support digestion. This is best done on an empty stomach, a few hours after eating. Start slowly and see how your body responds.

1. Lie on a comfortable floor mat or bed with your knees bent, feet flat on the surface below you.

2. Place your hand below your sternum, with your four fingers gentle pressing into your abdomen below either side of your rib cage.

3. Move your fingers in close clockwise circles, circling from just below your sternum and ribs down to your lower abdomen area below your belly button. Do this ten to twenty times, taking slow, deep breaths as you massage.

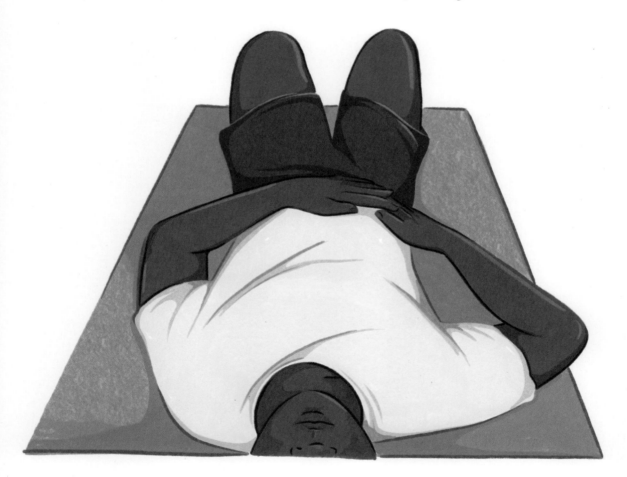

Vision Exercises

Exercises involving the visual system are some of the most impactful ways to quickly shift the state of your mind and body. Vision is the dominant sense that humans use to navigate the world, and there are very interesting bidirectional interactions between how we see and how we feel internally. Stress impacts the visual system, and intentionally engaging the visual system in specific ways can shift the body's stress response. I know this may be a new concept for many of you, so here are some quick eye facts:

- The muscles that hold your eyes in place are called your extraocular muscles and are the source of something called your ocular cardiac reflex. This reflex is mediated by the vagus nerve and is an immediate way to calm the body.

- Research estimates that 80 to 85 percent of our perception, learning, cognition, and activities are mediated through our vision.

- More than 50 percent of the cortex is devoted to processing visual information. More neurons are dedicated to vision than the other four senses combined.

- When the stress response is activated, pupils dilate, vision narrows in focus, and eyes dart from one place to the next; when feeling safe and connected, the opposite happens.

When the brain dedicates this much resourcing to something, we know it's really important. Your eyes and how you position and move them have a profound influence on the state of your brain.

Integrating the following exercises into your daily routine can help counteract some common ways that modern life negatively impacts our visual system. For example:

- Eye convergence (eyes moving together to focus on something up close) activates the sympathetic nervous system and decreases peripheral vision. This happens when we look at our phone or even a laptop screen.

- The fast-paced nature and high pressure of society today often creates chronic stress, causing us to spend more time in that tunnel vision state.

- Artificial blue light reaches further into the retina and can feel jarring to the nervous system (e.g., more pain, more fight-or-flight response). It also suppresses the production of melatonin—hence why so many research articles mention removing blue light exposure at least an hour before bed.

Eye movements increase blood flow to the vertebral artery and stimulate the vagus nerve as it passes through the upper neck. Stretching and relaxing muscles in the eye, and changing the way you are using your vision, can initiate a parasympathetic response and improve vagal activity. What I love most about vision exercises is that they are relatively quick and can be done almost anywhere.

Here are some vision therapy exercises to build into your day or in moments of stress to tip the scale back toward your parasympathetic nervous system state. Each of these can be done standing, seated, or lying on your back. In fact, you may even want to try switching up the position of your body as you do some of these to see whether one posture and exercise combination feels more supportive than another.

Lateral Eye Stretches

Eye movements have a direct connection to the suboccipital muscles that sit at the base of your skull. Laterally stretching your eyes reduces eyestrain and releases tight muscles in your neck to increase blood flow to the vagus nerve.

1. With your head facing forward and without moving it, move your eyes to the right for 30 to 90 seconds. You should be looking far enough to the right that you feel a gentle stretch but not so far that it feels like you're straining your eyes.

2. Take a moment to notice whether you have any signs of reset.

3. Repeat on the other side.

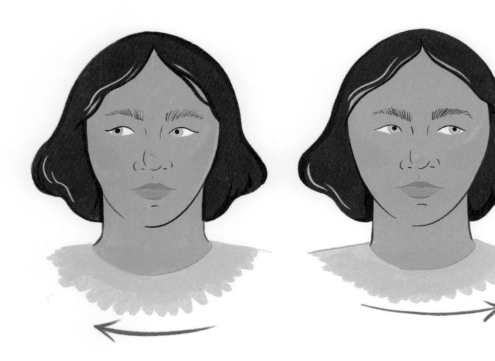

Eye Push-Ups

Eyes Converged

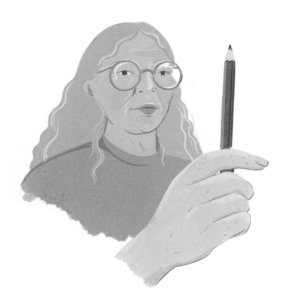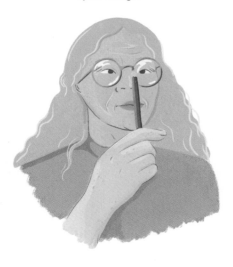

This exercise, also known as a near-far focusing exercise, helps reset the vagus nerve by alternating focus between objects at different distances. It can also improve eye coordination, reduce eyestrain, and encourage a release of the frequent eye convergence (which adds to physiological stress) that happens for many of us with frequent, close-up, daily phone and laptop use.

1. Hold a pen or your finger about 6 inches in front of your face and hold your eyes there for a couple of seconds until it comes into full focus.

2. Look through the pen to a point in the distance 10 or more feet away from you and hold your eyes on that point until it comes into clear focus, usually 1 to 2 seconds.

3. Return your eyes to focus on the pen close up and repeat, shifting your focus from the pen to the far away point for 1 to 2 minutes.

Orienting

Orienting is a way of nonverbally communicating to the nervous system that you are safe by better orienting to your surroundings.

1. Begin looking around you, moving your head and eyes freely as you slowly scan the space around you.

2. Notice whether your eyes are darting from one thing to the next: That's an indication you are in an active stress response. If that's the case, try to slow your eye scanning, making it as smooth and gentle as possible. Allow yourself to focus on one thing and then gently move to the next.

3. Do this for at least 30 seconds up to as long as you feel it is helpful.

Gaze Opening

As I previously mentioned, when you are in a stress response, your gaze narrows in focus. Gaze opening is when you intentionally widen that focus.

1. Without moving your head or eyes, try to bring more of your surroundings into focus.

2. Again, without moving your head or eyes, focus on your periphery. I will sometime place my hands about a foot away from my head on either side and wiggle my fingers to help my eyes expand focus to my peripheral vision.

Eye Cupping

This is also referred to as palming. It is an exercise to help relax the muscles around your eyes and reduce eye fatigue.

1. Rub your hands together to warm them up.

2. Cup your hands close to your eyes and rest the heels of your hands on the corresponding cheekbones covering each eye.

3. Stay in this position for 1 to 5 minutes. I often try to focus on taking deep breaths during this time as well.

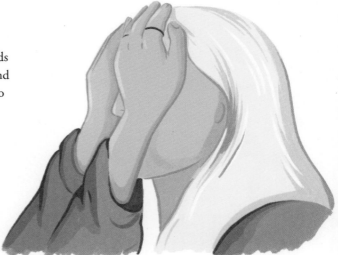

Distance Viewing

This is exactly what is sounds like. This isn't necessarily a specific exercise, but it felt important to note here that it is really beneficial and regulating to attempt to better balance out your close and distance viewing.

Try viewing things at a distance (out a window, across the room, or outside) for 10 to 20 minutes for every 90 minutes you have of close viewing (phone, laptop, writing).

Other Practices

Here are a variety of other research-supported practices that stimulate various branches of the vagus nerve, contributing to improvements in overall vagal tone.

Gargling, Humming, and Singing

The vagus nerve connects to your vocal cords and the muscles at the back of your throat. Activities like gargling, humming, and singing create vibrations and muscle contractions in this area that activate the vagus nerve and have been shown to improve heart rate variability. You know the yogi practice of chanting "om"—well, turns out that's particularly effective at calming and toning the vagus nerve. Not only does it vibrate the throat area, but the vibrations also extend up into the ear, where we have other vagus nerve connections. One study found that chanting "om" was helpful in deactivating certain parts of the limbic brain, like the amygdala, involved in stress and emotional responses. I love it when ancient wisdom meets modern science.

Keep these practices simple: Gargle for about 30 seconds in the morning and evening when you brush your teeth or when you're in the shower. Hum or sing in the shower or throughout your day, intuitively or intentionally, when you're feeling activated.

LAUGHTER AND SOCIALIZATION

We know that laughter and healthy socialization reduce stress hormones, and one way they likely do this is by activating the vagus nerve and shifting us more toward our parasympathetic state. Laughter physiologically engages the throat and abdomen muscles, both places where we find a lot of vagus nerve connections. General social connection also improves vagal tone through stress reduction, co-regulation, shared experiences, and emotional regulation. Researchers have even discovered that reflecting on positive social interactions can improve vagal tone and heart rate variability. Laughter and social connection seem to have a bidirectional relationship—the more you laugh and socialize, the higher your vagal tone; the higher your vagal tone, the more easily laughter and social connections come.

When you're feeling good, make a point to laugh often. Laugh with friends, laugh compassionately at yourself when you have one of those pesky human moments, or make it a point to consume funny content.

This may feel harder to do when you're not feeling so great, whether you are overwhelmed, anxious, or depressed. If that's the case, I still invite you in those moments to reach out to someone who feels supportive or watch something you'd usually find funny. It turns out you can even take on a "fake it 'til you make it" attitude with laughter. You can do a few big belly "HA HA HAs" and your body will stimulate the vagus nerve in a similar way.

Cold Exposure

Ice baths and cold showers have increased in popularity for good reason, as they have both physiological and psychological benefits. Studies show benefits that are far reaching, one of those being improved vagal tone and heart rate variability. Other positive physical side effects are improved immunity, improved metabolism, decreased stress, increased stress threshold, improved circulation, and reduced inflammation. Psychologically, with cold exposure you are consciously choosing to immerse yourself in something uncomfortable. You are resisting the urge to jump out or avoid it and instead you're staying with it and regulating through it. Thus, you're building your capacity for stress by being in a state where adrenaline levels are high but you're intentionally working to keep your mind calm. This is a meaningful and self-directed way to build resilience, grit, and impulse control. This can be a tough practice to get into. I don't know very many people who love being cold! But the benefits are huge and might be worth it for you.

Research suggests that deliberate cold exposure for approximately 11 minutes total per week is enough to optimize the benefits. This could look like two to four sessions, lasting 1 to 5 minutes each, spread out across the week. Like all the other practices in this book, this will look different from person to person.

The most common forms of cold exposure are ice baths or cold showers. Ice baths involve full body submersion into cold water while a cold shower is simply that: a really cold shower.

1. For an ice bath: Fill a bathtub or other container with cold water, adding ice to make it colder. For a cold shower: Turn on the shower as low as it will go (no ice is added to the shower).

2. Test the water temperature. You want it to be uncomfortably cold, meaning you feel like you really want to get out. But you also need to be able to safely stay in. This will vary from person to person and the experience you have with this practice. That specific temperature typically ranges from 60°F (15.5°C) for some down to 45°F (7.2°C) for others. Keep in mind that it seems that the colder the water the shorter amount of time you need to expose yourself for the maximum amount of benefits.

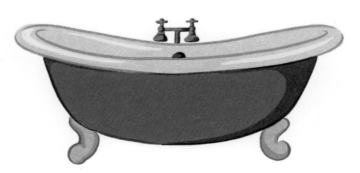

3. Get in the tub, submerging your body up to your neck, or hop in the cold shower. There will be an immediate shock, probably a sharp inhale, muscles tensing, and an urge to get out.

4. Breathe. At first, meet your system where it is with some short, quick breaths. Gradually work to slowing your breath and allowing your muscles to relax. The goal is to create a situation where you are uncomfortable (because of the cold) but calm.

5. Stay in for as long as you can, but don't exceed 15 minutes.

NOTE: When I first started ice baths and cold showers I was only able to stay in for about 30 seconds. I now tend to be in for about 5 minutes each session.

6. When your timer goes off, get out or turn the water off and let your body come back to a normal core temperature naturally—meaning to get the most out of this, don't immediately hop into a sauna or hot shower. Simply wrap yourself up in a towel or blanket, maybe drink a warm beverage, and allow your body temperature to naturally rise to normal.

NOTE: There is research that shows the benefits of hot/cold therapy wherein you alternate between an ice bath and sauna. This is a practice I personally do on occasion. Evidence for maximizing the benefits suggests starting in the hot and ending in the cold and then reheating naturally.

Another type of cold exposure is face immersion. Although it hasn't been found to have the broad-reaching mental and physical benefits of ice baths or cold showers, it can have profound impacts on an immediate acute stress response. This could be a practice to help pull you out of immediate moments of high anxiety or stress.

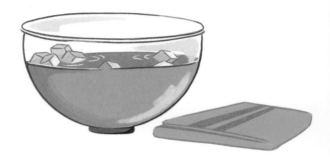

1. Fill a large bowl or sink with ice water.

2. Put your face (not your whole head, just your forehead, eyes, nose, cheeks, and chin) in the bowl of ice water for 5 to 30 seconds, or however long you are able to hold your breath.

3. Repeat one to three times.

Cold exposure can be a powerful tool for improving physical and mental health, but it should always be done safely and responsibly. It's important to note that everyone's body is different and there is no one-size-fits-all protocol to cold water therapy. In general, start mindfully and slowly when beginning cold exposure therapies. Gradually increase the exposure time and decrease the temperature. Listen to your body and stop if you experience any pain or concerning symptoms. If you have any preexisting medical conditions it's important to check with your doctor before starting cold exposure therapy.

YOGA

Yoga can be practiced in many ways, but in this context you are using it as a practice to promote mind-body connection by focusing on a few poses particularly supportive to the nervous system.

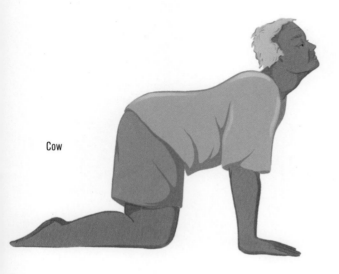

Cow

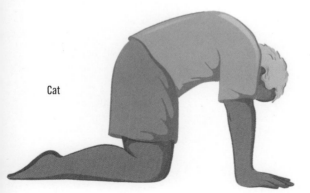

Cat

Cat Cow Transition

The vagus nerve extends down the spine and into the abdominal cavity. The transitional movement between cat post and cow pose mobilizes and provides movement to these areas.

1. Begin on your hands and knees, with your wrists directly under your shoulders and your knees directly under your hips.

2. Inhale slowly as you arch your back. Lift your head and tilt your tailbone toward the ceiling. This is the Cow Pose, with your belly dropping toward the floor, shoulder blades squeezing together.

3. Exhale slowly as you round your spine, tucking your chin toward your chest and pelvis forward. This is the Cat Pose, with your belly pulling toward your spine, shoulder blades far apart, and your back rounded like a scared cat.

4. Repeat this several times, continuing to move between Cow and Cat Pose, inhaling as you arch your back and exhaling as you round your spine.

You can even do this seated. Simply place your hands on your knees, then inhale, pushing your chest forward and arching your back. Pull your shoulders back and lift your chin. Exhale, tucking in your chin, rounding your shoulder forward, and rounding your back.

Mountain Pose

This pose promotes and trains good posture as well as active mind-body connection and groundedness.

1. Stand with your feet hip-width apart, distributing your weight evenly between both feet.

2. Extend your arms at your sides, palms forward, fingers actively extended. Focus on pulling your shoulders back and down.

3. Tuck your tailbone under and lengthen your spine.

4. Engage your leg muscles by pressing through the soles of your feet and gently flexing your quads, lifting your kneecaps.

5. Take slow, deep breaths and focus on remaining tall and open in this posture. Visualize yourself as a tall, strong mountain, grounded and stable.

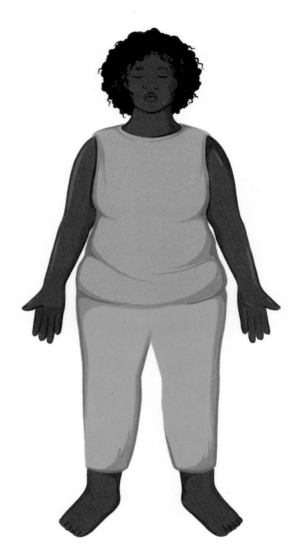

Legs Up the Wall

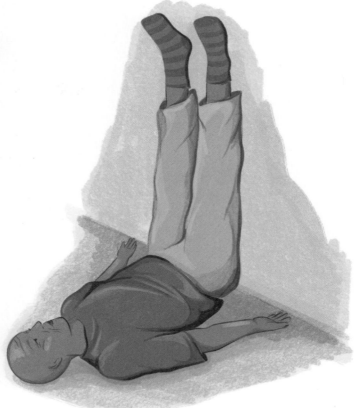

This is one of my favorites because it's so effective, simple, and well researched. It, along with the physiological sigh, are often some of the very first practices I invite my clients to implement. Resting in this gentle inverted position encourages your heart rate and breathing to slow, which then communicates to and through the vagus nerve that it is safe to start fully relaxing.

Previously in this book, I mentioned that changing the way you breathe can change your heart rate, and the reverse is true as well. When heart rate decreases, breath rate slows as well. In this pose, you'll use gravity to move some of the blood from your legs back toward your heart. With this extra blood flow, your heart doesn't have to work as hard, and your heart rate slows down, which in turn also slows down your breathing. Your heart and respiration are bidirectionally linked; understanding this is helpful because when you're in an activated state and want to down-regulate you can leverage either your respiration by deepening the breath and extending those exhales or your heart by using a pose like this to slow down your heart rate. So, if you're feeling anxious and can't catch your breath, try this pose to help you get there. Again, working *with* your physiology to impact your psychology is a powerful and tangible way to regulate your nervous system.

1. Find an open wall space. Sit as close as possible facing the wall.

2. Lower your shoulders and head to the floor, moving your legs up the wall.

3. Adjust your position by scooting your tailbone toward the wall. It doesn't need to touch the wall, but see how close you can get it while remaining comfortable.

4. Find a comfortable position for your arms to relax at your sides. Relax your legs against the wall. Settle into this pose and breathe for at least 2 minutes, increasing up to 15 minutes.

If this pose is uncomfortable, try a variation. Instead of putting your legs up the wall, place your heels on a chair, with your legs straight or knees bent at a 90-degree angle.

Yoga Nidra

This isn't a particular pose but a variation of yoga. Yoga nidra, also known as "yogic sleep," is a deeply restorative guided practice that helps reduce stress, anxiety, and tension in the body. During a yoga nidra practice, you recline or lie down in a comfortable position and follow a guided meditation that takes you through a series of visualization and relaxation techniques. Practices typically last from 20 to 40 minutes. This improves vagal tone by promoting relaxation, stimulating the parasympathetic nervous system, enhancing mind-body awareness, and reducing inflammation in the body. A similar practice is referred to as "non-sleep deep rest." You can find some great free guided sessions online.

Daily Movement or Exercise

Bodies are built to move. Regular movement and exercise are powerful tools for improving vagal tone. The specifics around what kind of movement or exercise don't seem to matter as much as the consistency of them. Whether it's aerobics, strength training, stretching, yoga, or tai chi, they all show positive impacts on vagal tone when consistently practiced. The exact amount for daily exercise needed to improve vagal tone can vary depending on things like age, fitness level, and overall health. Start where you are and build in more movement gradually. A sustainable and beneficial place for most of my clients is to build a habit of intentional movement or exercise practice 30 minutes a day four to five days a week.

Morning Sun Exposure

I recommend to all my clients the simple practice of spending about 10 minutes each morning sitting outside, letting natural sunlight into their eyes. The ideal amount time spent outside depends on how clear or cloudy the sky is. Just being outside is typically enough, but especially on cloudy days it can be beneficial to face the direction of the rising sun (without looking directly at the sun). Don't wear sunglasses (eyeglasses are fine) and stay off your phone.

This simple behavior has numerous mental and physical health benefits. It sets your circadian clock, promotes metabolic and hormone health, triggers a timed release of cortisol, which promotes wakefulness and focus throughout the day, and starts a timer for melatonin release later in the day, which supports better sleep. It's important to actually get outside for this practice or to view through an open window. Researchers say that windows filter out a lot of the blue light wavelengths that are essential for stimulating the eyes and this wake-up signal, making viewing the morning light through a window around fifty times less effective.

Smart Dietary Choices

The foods you consume impact your cellular and digestive health and inflammation levels. What you eat matters, but what that looks like is going to be different from person to person. Nutrition is highly personalized based on individual needs, preferences, and access. In general, avoid highly processed foods and try to incorporate as many seasonal fruits and vegetables as possible. Take specific note of probiotics and fiber, as they both support healthy gut microbiome and function, which contributes to reducing inflammation, regulating the immune system, enhancing neurotransmitter production, and improving overall well-being. This can come through supplementation or by consuming fibrous and fermented foods. I'm not going to spend any more time getting into the specifics because they're so unique to an individual. Keep it simple, make small shifts, and do your best to eventually get to a place where you are eating mostly healthy, most of the time.

Sleeping on Your Side

Research has found that lying on your back decreases heart rate variability (also indicating a decrease in vagal tone) while sleeping on your side increases vagus nerve stimulation. If you aren't already a side sleeper, I recommend placing a pillow between your knees while you sleep. This will help keep you from shifting onto your back or stomach as you sleep.

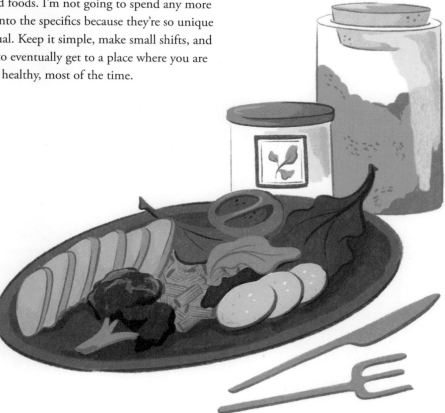

Practitioner- and Device-Supported Techniques

The previous techniques outlined ways you can stimulate the vagus nerve on your own. The following methods are ways you can get support from other practitioners or devices to activate the vagus nerve and improve overall vagal tone.

Auricular Acupuncture

Auricular acupuncture is a form of acupuncture that involves the stimulation of specific points on the ear. The vagus nerve mediates sensations of the outer ear, so using acupuncture here boosts the flow of information in the auricular branch of the vagus nerve, increasing overall activation.

Massage Therapy

Massage therapy can be a great tool for improving vagal tone because it promotes relaxation, reduces stress, and provides manual manipulation to soft tissues in the body. General massage techniques can be supportive, especially when the neck and shoulder areas are massaged. Other specific massage techniques that can be used to improve vagal tone are abdominal massage, craniosacral therapy, myofascial release, and reflexology. Reflexology, a type of massage the applies pressure to specific points on the feet, has been used to promote relaxation and stimulation of the nervous system, including the vagus nerve.

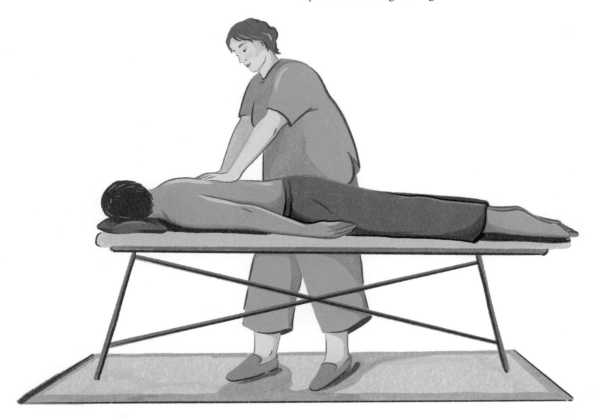

Chiropractic Care

Neck and back pain have become increasingly common as more and more jobs put us at a desk all day. Chiropractic care focuses on the treatment of the musculoskeletal system, particularly the spine. Research has shown that spinal cord stimulation by a chiropractor for individuals with neck or lower back pain significantly improves blood pressure and heart rate variability, increasing vagus nerve function. Reduction in chronic pain supports the nervous system in a shift toward a more parasympathetic state overall.

Electrical Stimulation

Electrical stimulation is a medical intervention to stimulate the vagus nerve. This involves an implanted device and is typically reserved for patients with severe treatment-resistant depression and/or epilepsy. There are other electrical stimulation devices that don't need to be implanted, but they show mixed results at the time of this writing. As tempting as electrical stimulation may sound as a passive means for improving vagal tone, I still recommend using daily exercises and forming supportive habits before trying external equipment like this.

Sensory Deprivation

Perhaps you've heard of a sensory deprivation tank, which is a specialized tank designed to decrease sensory input. This tank is typically a large, enclosed chamber filled with densely concentrated saltwater, which allows the body to float effortlessly. The tank is soundproof and completely dark, creating an environment that promotes a state of deep relaxation and inner focus (providing you do not suffer from claustrophobia). These are typically found at specific "float center" spas.

Visceral Manipulation

Visceral manipulation is a type of manual therapy that focuses on the manipulation, or gentle movement, of the internal organs and their surrounding connective tissues with the goal of improving the function of these organs and their structures. This can improve vagal tone by addressing areas that the vagus nerve innervates.

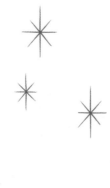

TOOLS FOR ACTIVATION (FIGHT-OR-FLIGHT)

You've heard me say multiple times throughout this book that different tools work better depending on which nervous system state you are in. This, and the following section, are designed to be a quick reference for some tools and practices that tend to be most supportive in regulating from a fight-or-flight state or a freeze/shutdown state. Note that these are mere suggestions; each individual must go on their own journey to identify which tools specifically support their nervous system in each state.

Note that you'll also discover that different tools are more supportive depending on the intensity of activation you are experiencing. For example, if you are feeling a lower intensity of activation, say a 1 to 5, then more gentle practices may be sufficient. On the other hand, if you are at a 6 to 10, then you'll need more mobilization. If you try to meditate while experiencing higher activation, it can actually increase dysregulation. Your system is essentially saying, "You didn't get the memo! It's not safe and we need to move!" Often the key in nervous system regulation is to first meet your nervous system *where it is* and then slowly shift it toward regulation. So when you are more highly activated, you want to do things that allow for more mobilization of your body first before doing anything too calm or still.

Let your body be the guide. These practices are designed to feel supportive. If they don't feel supportive for your system, listen to that and try another. Your body will tell you what feels helpful and right for you.

What to Look for When Regulating While in Activation

When in sympathetic activation, your system is primed to move, so part of regulating often involves *allowing* your body to move and discharge some of that excess energy, and then settle. You aren't looking to go from upregulated, angry, or anxious to immediately feeling regulated and great. Instead, you're looking for any amount of that sympathetic energy to discharge and leave your body. You want anything that helps you feel even a little bit more settled or calm, feel less tension and urgency, have clearer thinking, be less antsy, breathe more deeply, and have a slower heart rate.

Some tools I've already introduced that you may find supportive here are:

- Legs up the wall
- Extended exhale breath
- Ear or neck massage
- Orienting
- Gaze opening
- Eye cupping

There is no one magic tool either. Some tools work differently in different situations or at different levels of activation. You're looking to create a toolbox of practices that you can layer to help you regulate in these moments.

Additional Somatic Regulating Tools to Use When in Activation

The following tools are specifically designed to help decrease sympathetic activation. They are grouped in a suggestive way according to tools that tend to work best for my clients depending on the level of activation they are experiencing, low to moderate or moderate to high.

LEVEL OF ACTIVATION: 1 TO 5

The following exercises may help if you are experiencing a low to moderate amount of activation or anxiety.

Gentle Swaying or Stretching

Either seated or standing, allow your body to rock side to side or front to back. This repetitive and rhythmic motion is soothing to the nervous system. Gentle stretching also helps mobilize the body in a soothing way.

Box Breathing

1. Inhale deeply and fully through your nose for a count of 4.
2. Hold your breath at the top of the inhale for a count of 4.
3. Exhale slowly and fully through your mouth for a count of 4.
4. Hold your breath at the bottom of the exhale for a count of 4.
5. Repeat two to five times.

Color Spotting

Preemptively choose your "regulating color"—let's say it is orange. When you're feeling rising activation, pause to scan your surroundings. Count or name all the orange objects you can see. This acts as a way to temporarily distract you for what's creating the activation, orients you to your surroundings, and engages your visual system in a regulating way.

Tense and Release

Activation is preparing you to fight or run, and this tense and release practice allows you to lean into that urge and then invite it to soften. I often use this practice when I'm feeling the urgent need to control a situation.

1. Inhale as you tense all your muscles. Clench your fists, lift your shoulders, scrunch your face, flex your legs, and curl your toes.
2. Exhale as you release and relax everything.
3. Repeat a few times, until you notice it getting easier and easier to let go.

Heel Drops

1. Slowly raise yourself up onto your toes, then drop back onto your heels. Start with a smaller gentler lift and drop, finding a rhythm.

2. Build more height or speed, standing high on your tippy toes, and then letting yourself fall onto your heels, creating a "thud" sound.

3. Relax into the movement so you feel the reverberations through your body as you drop.

4. Continue for 1 minute.

Somatic Head Self-Holding Exercise

When your body is activated, your mind usually follows suit. If you're experiencing racing or catastrophizing thoughts, try somatic self-holding practices.

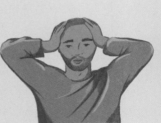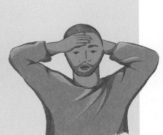

1. Place your hands on either side of your head or place one hand on your forehead and the other on the back of your head.

2. Feel the sensation between your hands. Notice how you are creating a container for your racing thoughts.

3. Take note whether your thoughts seem to slow and/or if this feels regulating or soothing for your system.

Somatic Shaking

Shaking is a way the body discharges activated stress energy, and it can be a way of completing a stress cycle and down-regulating. There's no right or wrong way to go about this, but here's some guidance to get started.

1. Stand up if you can and slowly begin to shake your hands, arms, and shoulders. I often start by shaking my hands like I'm trying to flick water off them. Allow the shaking to spread through your entire body. Start with gentle wiggling or shaking and gradually increase the intensity as you feel more comfortable.

2. Shake for 1 minute, focusing on releasing any tension or stress you may be holding in your body.

3. After a minute (or more if you'd like), slow down the shaking and bring it to a stop. Take a few moments to rest and notice how you're feeling.

Hold an Ice Cube or Suck on Sour Candy

As soon as you feel panic or intense activation coming on, close your palm around an ice cube or place a sour candy in your mouth. Focus on the intensity of the cold or tartness instead of trying to force stop your symptoms. These techniques are designed to jolt your system out of the fight-or-flight response by shocking the senses to distract from moments of high activation (e.g., panic).

Go for a Walk

This may feel like an obvious suggestion, but it bears including here as a reminder for a number of reasons. Walking puts your body in motion, allowing you to honor this state's need to mobilize. It also opens up your vision and makes you more aware of your surroundings, all shifting you toward the parasympathetic state. It's also easy to tool layer here. While walking you can get outside, focus on your breath, do some distance viewing, or do somatic shaking.

TOOLS FOR SHUTDOWN AND FREEZE

These states are *protective* mechanisms for when stressors get too big or last too long. This state's two goals are to conserve energy through immobilization and to prevent further pain through numbing and disconnection. Therefore, regulation happens by gently inviting connection and mobilization to your system. In freeze your system is so overwhelmed that it gets "frozen" or stuck, creating immobilization. When in dorsal vagal shutdown, you can think about it like a bear in hibernation: Your system is essentially shutting off. With both these states if you bring too much energy into the system at once you may reinforce the need to stay stuck and shut down. Think about these states like a Chinese finger trap: The harder you pull or force, the more stuck you become.

The goal isn't to bounce from feeling overwhelmed, stuck, numb, flat, disconnected, or depressed right into feeling regulated. When regulating, you need to meet your system where it is first and then slowly walk it toward regulation. As you just read about with the sympathetic activation state, you need to meet that state *in* mobilization first. The more activated you feel, the more mobilization or intensity you need to allow at first, and then slowly step toward being more still and calm.

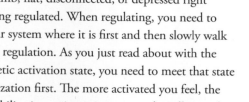

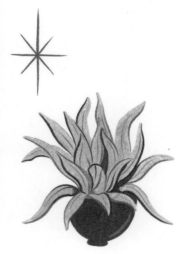

When in shutdown or freeze, the same applies but in the opposite direction. The more shut down you are, the more gently you need to invite in the connection and mobilizing energy.

One other note on shifting out of shutdown and freeze is that when regulating from these states it can be common for symptoms to shift from being shut down and disconnected to feeling activated or anxious. When my clients first experience this they assume something has gone wrong but, in fact, it's quite the opposite. Remember those nervous system zones? When regulating from a shutdown state (aka red zone), you must move *through* mobilization (aka yellow zone) on the way up to regulation. This is another important place where tool layering comes in. You'll have tools for when you're shut down and then when that state loosens its grip and new sensations of activation arise, you'll shift into using tools from your activation toolbox to regulate from there.

Let your body be the guide and know that there is always another practice to try if what you're doing doesn't feel supportive.

What to Look for When Regulating While in Shutdown or Freeze

When in these states, your system is "stuck" or "frozen." This happens when the threat seems too big or has lasted too long and you no longer believe you can cope. You're looking to get that shutdown or frozen experience to loosen up just a bit—think about coming out of these states like a bear coming out of hibernation, slow and steady. You're looking for anything that helps you notice your body more, be more awake or energized, feel more connected or present, have clearer thinking, breathe more deeply, or notice your senses more fully.

Some tools I've already introduced that you may find supportive here are:

- Diaphragmatic breathing
- "Voo" breath
- Ear or neck massage
- Eye stretches
- Orienting
- Cold exposure
- Humming
- Laughter and socialization (coregulation)

Additional Regulating Tools to Use When in Shutdown or Freeze

The following tools are specifically designed to help you activate from a shutdown or frozen state.

Intentional Rest or Disconnection

The goal isn't always to fix; sometimes the down time this state creates is effective (if you surrender to it with intention). So often we find ourselves in a shutdown state but continue to force more going and doing. Even though it sounds counterintuitive, meeting your system in and facilitating the need for immobilization and disconnection might be the most helpful thing you can do and can create natural capacity to reconnect and mobilize. It's not that disconnection and immobilization are bad; it's how often and in what ways you engage them.

1. Try to consciously recognize the next time you're in the red zone and understand that the intention of this state is to disconnect and conserve energy.

2. Think: How can I do this intentionally? It might be to scroll on your phone, watch a show, or go lay in bed. These might be things you currently do *unintentionally* to zone out or numb. The key is to simply build awareness and intention around what's happening and to allow your system the *temporary* rest and disconnection it needs to be able to come back online naturally.

Single Task Action

Choose a task that you can complete and mobilize around—something like doing the dishes, running an errand, getting up to get a glass of water, or writing a single email. Choose a task that feels small and manageable for the state you are in. This could even be something as simple as changing your location. Stuck in bed? Move to the couch. Zoning out on the couch? Go sit on the porch. This small act of moving or doing begins to reverse the spiral of shutdown.

Listen to Music

While doing so, hum or sing along. Listening engages our hearing sense and humming or singing along activates the vagus nerve.

Experience Temperature Change

These practices bring you back into connection with your body and the present moment. You can do this by:

- Running your hands under cold or warm water, noticing the temperature and sensation as you do

- Taking a cold shower

- Eating frozen fruit

- Going outside

Sensory Awareness

Look around you and notice:

- 5 things you can see

- 4 things you can feel

- 3 things you can hear

- 2 things you can smell

- 1 thing you can taste

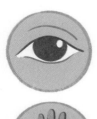

Sliding out of the shutdown or frozen state is a gentle process. The key is to connect to your body and senses.

Sharp Breathing

This is an upregulating breath practice. These sharp inhales and exhales shift your physiology, inviting activation into your system, making it less comfortable to remain still or frozen. Experiment with this practice slowly, especially when in a freeze state, because you don't want to further overload your system. You can adjust or moderate the intensity of this breath practice in a number of ways as well.

1. Take a few deep breaths to connect to your breath.

2. Sharply inhale through your nose for a count of 1. Feel your rib cage expand.

3. Sharply exhale through your mouth for a count of 1. Feel your abdomen contract and push the air out.

4. Continue to quickly transition between quick inhales and exhales for up to a minute. You may notice your heart rate increase and energy begin to pulse through your body. The goal is to make it uncomfortable to stay immobilized but not to be overwhelming for your system.

Somatic Posture Change

People in a shutdown or frozen state often embody a collapsed posture, trying to get small, surrender, or disappear. Follow these steps to allows you to lean into that urge and then invite your body into a more open and able posture.

1. While seated, collapse your posture, allow yourself to slump over, and hang your head and arms toward or between your knees.

2. As you inhale, slowly roll your spine upright, one vertebrae at a time, letting your head be the last thing to rise, until you are sitting up straight.

3. Then begin to stand up, slowly. Once you're standing all the way up, pull your shoulders back, puffing out your chest.

4. Notice how it feels to stand in more power, to take up more space.

5. Repeat as needed.

Gentle Body Squeeze

When in a shutdown or frozen state, it's common to become disconnected from your body, experiencing things like dissociation or depersonalization. This practice gently invites you back into awareness of and connection with your body using neutral or pleasurable sensations, which read as safe to the nervous system.

1. Cross your arms like you're going to give yourself a hug, placing your hands on the opposite shoulder.

2. Gently squeeze your shoulders and continue to move your hands down your arms, providing gentle and nurturing squeezes. You can also repeat in your mind, "These are my arms."

3. Continue this practice with any other part of your body. Gently squeeze or rub different body parts and repeat in your mind, "This is my neck/chest/legs."

4. Pause to notice how you're feeling and whether there's any other body part that you could connect to.

The final chapter of this book provides suggested blueprints on how you can work these various tools and practices into your everyday life to help you tap into the healing power of the vagus nerve.

QUICK SUMMARY

- Vagal tone improves anytime the vagus nerve is activated or you move toward a more regulated nervous system state in any way.

- Vagal toning exercises only work to improve vagal tone when practiced consistently over a period of time.

- Somatic practices encompass a broader range of techniques aimed at addressing the mind-body connection, releasing physical tension, and healing trauma.

- When trying new tools, you can follow the simple framework to assess, practice, and reassess to note the effectiveness of a tool in the moment.

- Different tools work for different nervous system states. Through experimentation, you'll cultivate a regulation toolbox that is unique to and effective for you.

7

CREATING A VAGAL TONING ROUTINE

Changing your life means changing something you do daily. Healing lies in your daily routine.

Improved vagal tone happens when you build these tools into your daily life. After everything we've talked about so far, it's natural to have questions like, "Where do I start?" or "How do I even begin to put it all together?" I've got you covered! That's exactly the work I support my clients in every day and what I'm going to walk you through in this chapter. The short answer to those questions is that you're going to start where you are, with the current capacity you have. Start small, installing one tiny habit at a time, and then optimize it little by little. It will eventually come together, adapting to the various seasons of your life.

One thing I commonly hear at this point is, "I logically *know* the things I should be doing, but I can't seem to get myself to actually *do* them." This often happens when you try to shoot for an "ideal" routine when your capacity doesn't match that. Behavior change, installing new habits, takes time and intention, but it is absolutely possible! It can also be incredibly helpful to seek out support on this journey to creating healthier habits.

ESTABLISHING A ROUTINE

When it comes to building new routines, it's helpful to remember that habit change can be hard, especially when you're currently living with a dysregulated nervous system. The whole point of this new routine is that it happens on a regular basis. If you try to do too much, too soon, it'll just add stress to your system and reinforce dysregulation. I know it sounds cliché but think about this like a marathon, not a sprint. Healing, regulating, and improving vagal tone is a lifelong journey. I think you'll find when you can ditch the urgency and rush, and instead begin celebrating the small steps and changes along the way, they will add up in transformational ways.

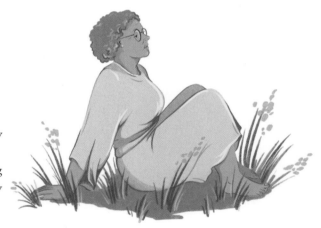

When choosing a new habit, many people ask themselves, "What can I do on my best days?" The trick for sustainable habit change is to instead ask, "What can I still stick to even on my worst days?" In other words, install tiny habits and then scale up from there as your capacity and confidence increase. Start by adding one or two simple practices from chapter 6 to your life, maybe something like gargling after brushing your teeth or humming in the shower. At first this may feel insignificant and unimpactful, but each time you engage these practices you are stimulating your vagus nerve more than you were before in a way that doesn't add stress load to your nervous system. Now, it'll obviously take more than daily gargling or humming to see a noticeable difference in vagal tone, but this is a simple place to start that does make a difference and acts as a springboard for incorporating other habits.

To help my clients answer the question "Where do I start?" we work together to answer these questions:

1. What's your number one proactive self-care habit? Now, what's the smallest step you can take in improving that?

2. What practice feels the easiest for you to incorporate right now?

This helps people identify what matters most and what they could likely stick to, even on their worst days. I then support clients in taking tangible action to build in tiny, seemingly insignificant habits, celebrating the heck out of every little action. Then, with repetition and time, they build toward more optimal routines and practices. Let's walk through some of this same exploration together to help you get an idea of where you might like to start and what this could look like for you.

Exploring Your Unique Routine

These questions will help you figure out where to start in creating a vagal toning routine. Take some time to reflect on these questions—maybe even grab a journal and write it out.

1. What is your number one self-care habit?

   a. What is the number one thing that when it happens consistently you feel better—less anxious, calmer, and more capable. Overall, your unwanted symptoms decrease, and you have an increased capacity to handle more of life. (It could be sleep, movement, nutrition, social connection, etc.)

   b. What does that habit look like now?

   c. What would the ideal version of that habit look like?

   d. Now, what is the smallest change you can make stepping from where you currently are with this lifestyle habit toward where you'd like to be instead?

   e. How can you make that change even tinier?

   I will add that for most my clients their number one answer is sleep. Research supports this is most people's most impactful lifestyle habit. So if you're not sure where to start, start there. Optimizing your sleep has the most significant ripple effect in supporting every other psychological and physiological function.

2. What practice feels the easiest for you to incorporate right now?

   a. Review some of the vagal toning practices in the last chapter. What feels easy?

   b. Which practice do you think you could incorporate even on your most stressful or overwhelming days?

   c. What does it look like for you to integrate this into your daily life?

   d. What might get in the way of that? How can you overcome that?

   e. How do you feel when you think about incorporating this into your daily life? (If you feel at all overwhelmed by it, then choose a different practice or make this practice even easier.)

   These questions should help you establish a starting point for building vagal toning practices into your life. Once those small shifts become your new normal, you can ask variations of these questions again.

3. What would be another way to move closer to your ideal number one self-care habit?

4. Once that habit gets to a supportive and stable place, what's your number two self-care habit and how can you take a tiny step toward a more helpful baseline there?

5. What other practices feel easy or like they would make a difference for you? What does incorporating that into your daily life now look like?

   As you do this, slowly layering on one habit after the other, you will improve vagal tone and create a different, more supportive, and healed life for yourself.

ROUTINE BLUEPRINT EXAMPLES

You didn't think I was just going to leave you hanging out there in the theoretical to figure this all out on your own, did you? Those questions are powerful in determining where to start, but I also know it can be helpful to have a blueprint. I want to be clear that what I'm about to offer you is a *general* blueprint, not a universal protocol that *should* be followed. I firmly believe in personalization of behavior change in just about every step of someone's healing journey. This is why I think coaching is such a powerful resource, because it allows for real-time support, feedback, and adjustments. Consider this blueprint as a mere suggestion and give yourself permission to adjust and adapt it to better meet your needs, preferences, and the unique circumstances of your current life in any way you see fit.

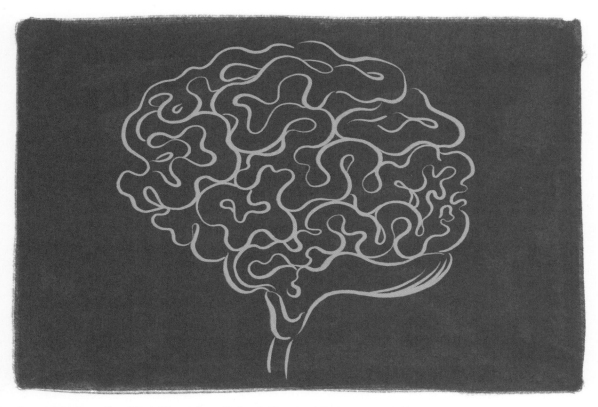

Everyone's healing routine will look different. Generally, though, it's easiest to implement a new habit by attaching it to a preexisting one. Then, in each new phase, continue integrating new habits.

This blueprint has four phases. Each phase is broken up into an a.m. and a p.m. sequence. I find that most of my clients have the most control over the first and last ten to fifteen minutes of their day. If building these habits during different parts of your day works better for you, you have unconditional permission to adjust and adapt.

I also recommend, as often as possible, to attach these new habits to habits or behaviors you already have. The existing habit becomes a cue, or a reminder, to do the new habit. For example, you might add gargling for thirty seconds after you brush your teeth, or you might start intentionally humming in the shower, or you may decide while using the toilet throughout the day that you will do a nervous system check-in or practice a few diaphragmatic breaths.

Plan to concentrate on each phase for anywhere from two weeks to a few months depending on how long it takes you to make that your new norm. There is no timeline, and there is no rush. You want the phase you're in to become easy, automatic, and habitual before adding more. Also note that it's okay if these phases don't happen perfectly linearly. You may make it to phase 3 and then life hands you something hard. Your capacity must shift to deal with that thing and you notice the extra habits from phase 3 aren't happening. Instead of feeling like a failure, recognize how perfectly human this is, step back to phase 2, and remember that anything extra is something you can celebrate instead of feeling frustrated when it doesn't happen perfectly.

Phase 1 Blueprint

New Habits: Gargling and Diaphragmatic Breathing

At this point your routine looks something like this:

A.M.:

- 30 seconds of gargling

P.M.:

- 30 seconds of gargling and 1 to 5 minutes of intentional diaphragmatic breathing

TIPS: Instead of a quick rinse and spit after brushing your teeth, simply extend the practice out by 30 seconds to include gargling. The 1 to 5 minutes of intentional diaphragmatic breathing is to help build breath awareness and activate the vagus nerve—this can be done during any part of your day but might be most helpful to do just before or as you first lie down in bed to go to sleep.

Phase 2 Blueprint

Continue Integrating: Gargling and Diaphragmatic Breathing

New Habits: Morning Sunlight and "Voo" Breaths

At this point your routine looks something like this:

A.M.:

- 30 seconds of gargling

- 5 to 10 minutes outside, allowing that morning light into your eyes. Do a few "voo" breaths while outside.

P.M.:

- 30 seconds of gargling

- 1 to 5 minutes of diaphragmatic as you are preparing for sleep

TIPS: I'm a big fan of tool layering, so why not get sunlight and do your "voo" breaths at the same time? You could swap out "voo" breaths for any of the vision therapy exercises or simply do focused diaphragmatic breathing. Experiment with what works best for you.

Phase 3 Blueprint

Continue Integrating: Gargling, Diaphragmatic Breathing, Morning Sunlight, and "Voo" Breaths

New Habits: Legs Up the Wall and Eye Stretches

At this point your routine looks something like this:

A.M.:

- 30 seconds of gargling

- 5 to 10 minutes outside. Do a few "voo" breaths while outside.

P.M.:

- 30 seconds of gargling

- 3 to 10 minutes of legs up the wall; while there focus on diaphragmatic breathing and do one to three rounds of lateral eye stretches

TIPS: I love legs up the wall at night because it helps calm my system after a busy day to prepare for a better night's sleep. Again, you'll see more tool layering here. Let's heal smarter, not harder.

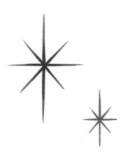
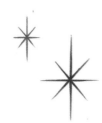

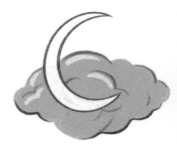

Phase 4 Blueprint

Continue Integrating: Gargling, Diaphragmatic Breathing, Morning Sunlight, "Voo" Breaths, Legs Up the Wall, and Eye Stretches

New Habits: Movement and Massage

Here are two variations of this routine, switching up the how and when to incorporate movement.

VERSION 1: Morning Movement

A.M.:

- 30 seconds of gargling

- 5- to 10-minute brisk walk outside; this incorporates your morning sunlight and movement, and you can even add in your "voo" breaths as well

P.M.:

- 30 seconds of gargling

- 1 to 2 minutes each side of a vagal toning ear and/or neck massage

- 3 to 10 minutes of legs up the wall; while there focus on diaphragmatic breathing and do one to three rounds of lateral eye stretches

VERSION 2: Evening Movement

A.M.:

- 30 seconds of gargling

- 5 to 10 minutes outside; also do a few "voo" breaths and a vagal toning ear and/or neck massage while outside

P.M.:

- 30 seconds of gargling

- 5 minutes of somatic shaking, swaying, and/or stretching

- 3 to 10 minutes of legs up the wall; while there focus on diaphragmatic breathing and do one to three rounds of lateral eye stretches

TIPS: Adding movement to your daily routine can look a million different ways. The goal here is to simply be intentional about *something* for 5 to 10 minutes a day. Maybe you already have an exercise habit. If so, great! Maybe instead of walking in the morning you just want to be outside and stretch. Go for it! Find a way to connect with your body that feels supportive and regulating.

What I love about this is that even at phase 4, no part of your a.m. or p.m. routine takes more than 5 to 15 minutes. And on any day that you're rushed and can't even spare 5 minutes, scale it back down to just gargling or any other single practice. The key here is to ditch the rigid perfectionism and instead remember that something is better than nothing. Consistent "somethings" are what add up to change everything.

Along the way, in addition to building your proactive vagal toning routine, I hope you're also experimenting with some reactive tools that help you regulate in moments of activation or shutdown. It's the combination of proactive routines and the use of regulation tools in real time that creates a powerful shift in healing.

LIVING A HEALING LIFE

The reality is that you can do all the vagal toning exercises in the world, but if your overall lifestyle is still fueling dysregulation and chronic stress, then there's only so much healing that can happen. The exercises are still helpful, but they can only do so much if you're still living in chronic survival mode. It's like having a sprained ankle, then wearing an ankle brace but continuing to run on it every morning. Wearing the ankle brace is supportive, but your ankle is going to have a hard time doing any kind of productive healing if you're continuing to stress it each day by running.

The same applies to your nervous system. Regulation comes from cultivating supportive practices, stress management, and intentional lifestyle shifts—gradually, strategically, and consistently applied. Let's explore what it looks like to live a healing life by combining proactive and reactive tools.

Bringing Together Proactive and Reactive Tools

First, a quick refresher is in order.

Proactive Tools: These are the consistent habits or lifestyle practices, done proactively, to improve vagal tone and create a life more suited for nervous system regulation. This includes your vagal toning routines, lifestyle changes, stress management, and deeper healing work. These increase your capacity to handle life's load and lay down new patterns for your future behaviors and reactions.

Occasionally revisit the proactive habits chart on pages 92 and 93 to assess how each of those categories is going for you. If there's one that feels particularly unmanaged, focus on small aspects you might be able to shift in a more supportive way.

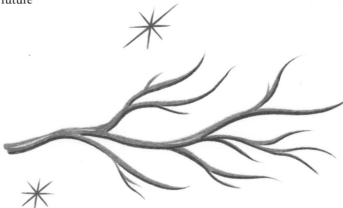

Reactive Tools: These are the *in-the-moment* regulation tools and practices that help you reverse the spiral of activation or shutdown. Some of these tools may be the same as the proactive vagal toning practices; here you just use them in response to moments of dysregulation. This also includes a variety of somatic and emotional regulation tools.

Remember on pages 58 and 59 where you learned how to map out your nervous system? You cultivated more awareness by exploring the different states with their specific sensations, emotions, thoughts, and behaviors for each. Then, beginning on page 126, I shared some tools that tend to work better depending on whether you're in activation or shutdown. Bringing both of those pieces together, you can begin to map out the reactive regulating tools that work best for you in each state. I call this a "Regulation Game Plan." It might look something like this:

REGULATION GAME PLAN

State: _____

	What is it like for me to be mildly, moderately, or very activated or shut down? SENSATIONS, EMOTIONS, THOUGHTS, BEHAVIORS	What reactive tools help me to regulate when I am in this place? TOOLS, STRATEGIES, RESOURCES
1		
2		
3		

There are no firm rules for how you combine reactive and proactive tools and practices. It's like a dance. And just like dancing, the more rigid you become about it, the harder it gets. Allow space for your humanness. Get curious and adopt an experimenter's mindset. Try something just to see whether it works. If it's supportive, keep doing it. If it's not, try something different. If you're feeling frustrated or overwhelmed, seek out support.

You'll adjust these routines countless times as you discover what the best fit is for your nervous system and daily life. One of the things I love so much about these tools is that they are simple, quick, and work with your physiology in tangible ways. I often refer to them as "micro moments of self-care." At least 752 times someone has told me, "I don't have time for self-care." My response is always the same: "You don't have time NOT to do self-care and I promise there are micro self-care practices that can fit into even the most stressful and busy days." As I mentioned, even phase 4 doesn't take more that 5 to 15 minutes on the bookends of your day. This is the work I specialize in—helping people create a personalized healing protocol that fits into whatever their current capacity is or their current season of life allows. These protocols are built on the foundation of my clients understanding of how their nervous system operates so that they can work with it in tangible, small, and powerful ways to support their healing. I see this work powerfully transform lives every day, and I know it can work for you too.

Daily, Weekly, and Occasional Practices

Consider a framework for establishing which practices you'd like to incorporate and at what frequency. Not all the tools suggested up to this point are meant to be incorporated in daily. Some may be more realistic or beneficial to do weekly, or occasionally. Specifics of this take some time and tweaking based on your unique needs, capacity, resources, and lifestyle, but as you step into this work of collecting regulation reps it can be helpful to categorize practices. I have clients establish practices that happen daily, weekly, monthly, and occasionally/as needed as "daily practices," "weekly practices," and "occasional practices."

Remember, the goal is not to do all the practices or try to incorporate all the new habits overnight (or even ever). Instead, focus on choosing one, make it a habit, then choose another, slowly layering one new habit on top of the other.

COMPASSION, CURIOSITY, AND CO-REGULATION

Three qualities to cultivate on this journey are compassion, curiosity, and co-regulation. On my own personal journey, I have found a deep sense of compassion for myself as I've come to better understand my nervous system, and I see the same happening daily for my clients. The key is to lean into the truth that in any given moment you're doing the best you can based on the current state of your nervous system, past lived experiences, and the tools that you have. For example, when I get snappy at my kid, or overreact in a situation, I rarely beat myself up about it anymore. I no longer fuel the narrative that "I'm a bad mom" or "too dramatic"— I know these are all signs I'm dysregulated and need to turn to my toolbox.

A client shared another work-related example of this when they realized how anxious they were after a particular meeting at work where they stated an opinion that not everyone agreed with. Instead of the old narrative of "You're an idiot, you shouldn't have said anything. Go fix it or just get over it," they were able to notice the activation in their system, take a quick pause, and notice their thoughts instead sounded like, "Makes sense you're feeling uneasy about how that went. Go take a walk, shake it off, it'll work out." They noticed their body's signals and instead of invalidating and dismissing these feelings they were able to acknowledge and validate them and then take tangible action to help their system soothe and regulate.

These moments also allow you to practice curiosity. You can turn inward and ask yourself, "What's up? What's contributing to my dysregulation right now? What might have just been triggering? What would I like to do about it?" This helps keep you in the driver's seat of your mind, body, and life in an empowering way.

Then there's co-regulation. I spent most of my teenage years and early adulthood developing a fierce and toxic independence. I didn't need help; I was always the helper. If I wanted it done "right," I did it myself. I developed debilitating productivity-based self-worth and did all the things all the time until it crushed me. I see this a lot in the clients I work with now as well. The reality is, we need each other. As humans, we are hardwired for connection. It is okay, and totally normal, that sometimes you can't regulate on your own. It's so important to get professional help when you need it.

QUICK SUMMARY

- Build routines around tiny habits that can survive even your worst days.

- Not sure where to start? Get clear on what matters most and what feels the easiest right now. As your capacity and confidence grow, so can your routines.

- There is no timeline or rush when it comes to building these practices into your life. Your goal is to have these habits for the rest of your life, so who cares how long it takes? Stay committed to something consistently while also allowing yourself to be a human that ebbs and flows based on what's going on in your life.

- Compassion, curiosity, and co-regulation are the magic ingredients to healing. Make space for your humanness and keep trying until you find the right fit. Working with a practitioner to support and guide you in this process can be incredibly beneficial.

FINAL THOUGHTS

From the beginning of this book, I've shared with you that my goal was to provide you with much more than a scientific understanding of your vagus nerve or a list of "vagus nerve hacks." I wanted to help you build an understanding of, and relationship with, your entire nervous system in a way that feels tangible and applicable to your healing journey. There is no one-size-fits-all blueprint to improving vagal tone or healing things like anxiety, depression, or chronic illness. But there are powerful research-supported practices that can help you work with your physiology to shift and heal your psychology in measurable and tangible ways. I've shared many of those with you here. It is now your job to put those pieces together in a way that creates your unique path to healing.

I truly believe in your capacity to heal. I don't believe you, or anyone, is born broken. I think throughout our lives we (and our nervous systems) have had to come up with countless creative ways to get our needs met, find belonging, and survive. I think we have all endured some terribly hard things that no one prepared us for. Many of us had loving and supportive parents, but just as many of us did not, and we're all here as adults learning how to self-regulate and heal to break out of these unhelpful patterns and create the beautiful lives we want.

You are doing the best you can based on your lived experiences, your current life circumstances, and the tools you have right now. I'm so proud of you for picking up a book like this and seeking out healing. You have everything you need to heal already inside of you, and it's okay that healing doesn't happen on your own (it's not meant to). Just like an athlete already has everything inside themselves to accomplish amazing things, they still need a coach to provide experience, strategy, training, and encouragement to help them get there. Please don't shy away from seeking out support on your healing journey.

What I've offered you in this book, and what I offer my clients daily, are the education, tools, strategy, and support I wish I had earlier in my own healing journey. But what I want you to get most out of this book is a sense of hope. Hope in healing. Hope in a way forward that puts you back in the driver's seat of your mind, body, and life. You can improve vagal tone and regulate your nervous system, and with that your entire life can change. Nervous system regulation is the foundation of all other healing.

There is no right or wrong way to go about this work. There is no rush or timeline to follow. It looks the way it will look and takes as long as it takes. Healing is going to have highs and lows. It will never be linear, but it is always in some way moving you forward. Different seasons of life will call for different approaches. Different capacities lend themselves to different actions. Take your time, make space for your humanness, find support, follow the guidelines given in this book, and in time you'll be able to look back in wonder at how far you've come.

RESOURCES

Book Recommendations

Accessing the Healing Power of the Vagus Nerve: Self-Help Exercises for Anxiety, Depression, Trauma, and Autism, by Stanley Rosenberg. This book offers insights into the role of the vagus nerve in regulating the nervous system and provides practical exercises for promoting vagal tone and healing from trauma.

The Anatomy of Anxiety, by Ellen Vora. This book is a comprehensive guide that explores the underlying causes of anxiety and provides a holistic approach to managing it through lifestyle and environmental factors, and promoting emotional well-being through a combination of traditional and alternative therapies.

Anchored: How to Befriend Your Nervous System Using Polyvagal Theory, by Deborah Dana. This book draws on the principles of polyvagal theory to offer a somatic approach to healing and practical strategies for regulating the nervous system through the development of resilience and social engagement.

Atomic Habits: An Easy & Proven Way to Build Good Habits & Break Bad Ones, by James Clear. This book provides a step-by-step approach to building and maintaining new habits, with practical strategies for overcoming obstacles and making lasting changes.

The Body Keeps the Score: Brain, Mind, and Body in the Healing of Trauma, by Bessel van der Kolk. This book explores how trauma affects the body and nervous system, and provides insights into the latest research on trauma therapy.

Bouncing Back: Rewiring Your Brain for Maximum Resilience and Well-Being, by Linda Graham. This book offers insights into the neurobiology of resilience and provides practical strategies for cultivating resilience in the face of adversity and trauma.

The Brain's Way of Healing: Remarkable Discoveries and Recoveries from the Frontiers of Neuroplasticity, by Norman Doidge. This book lays out the latest research on neuroplasticity and the brain's ability to heal itself while providing insights into innovative therapies and techniques that harness the brain's natural healing capacity to treat a range of conditions, from chronic pain to traumatic brain injury.

Breath: The New Science of a Lost Art, by James Nestor. This book explores the science and history of breathwork, and provides insights into how breathwork can regulate the nervous system, promote health, and enhance well-being.

The Complex PTSD Workbook: A Mind-Body Approach to Regaining Emotional Control and Becoming Whole, by Arielle Schwartz. This workbook offers a step-by-step approach to healing from complex trauma, incorporating both cognitive and somatic techniques.

The Healing Power of the Breath: Simple Techniques to Reduce Stress and Anxiety, Enhance Concentration, and Balance Your Emotions, by Richard P. Brown and Patricia L. Gerbarg. This book explores the role of breathwork in promoting vagal tone and regulating the nervous system, and provides practical exercises for improving mental health and well-being.

Healing Trauma: A Pioneering Program for Restoring the Wisdom of Your Body, by Peter A. Levine and Ann Frederick. This book provides a detailed guide to somatic experiencing, a therapy approach that focuses on the body's innate healing capacity.

The Mind-Gut Connection: How the Hidden Conversation within Our Bodies Impacts Our Mood, Our Choices, and Our Overall Health, by Emeran Mayer. This book lays out the relationship between the gut and the nervous system, and how the vagus nerve plays a crucial role in regulating digestion, mood, and overall health.

The Myth of Normal: Trauma, Illness, and Healing in a Toxic Culture, by Gabor Maté. This book challenges the concept of "normality" in mental health and the stigma surrounding mental illness. It argues that the current state of our society creates and perpetuates mental health struggles and provides suggestions for health and healing.

No Bad Parts: Healing Trauma and Restoring Wholeness with the Internal Family Systems Model, by Richard C. Schwartz. This book explores the internal family systems (IFS) model of therapy, which views the mind as a system of different parts. The book provides practical strategies for using the IFS model to heal trauma and restore wholeness, with a focus on self-compassion and developing a sense of internal safety.

Nurturing Resilience: Helping Clients Move Forward from Developmental Trauma—An Integrative Somatic Approach, by Kathy L. Kain and Stephen J. Terrell. This book offers a somatic approach to healing from developmental trauma, incorporating techniques for regulating the nervous system and promoting vagal tone.

Our Polyvagal World: How Safety and Trauma Change Us, by Stephen W. Porges and Seth Porges. This book presents the polyvagal theory in a way that is understandable to all and demonstrates how its practical principles are applicable to anyone looking to live their safest, healthiest, and happiest life.

The Polyvagal Theory: Neurophysiological Foundations of Emotions, Attachment, Communication, and Self-Regulation, by Stephen W. Porges. This book delves into the polyvagal theory, a neurobiological model of human behavior and emotions, and offers insights into the relationship between the nervous system, social engagement, and mental health.

Rewire Your Anxious Brain: How to Use the Neuroscience of Fear to End Anxiety, Panic, and Worry, by Catherine M. Pittman and Elizabeth M. Karle. This book offers a neuroscience-based approach to managing anxiety, with practical strategies for rewiring the brain and overcoming negative thought patterns.

Scattered Minds: The Origins and Healing of Attention Deficit Disorder, by Gabor Maté. This book explores the impact of attention deficit hyperactivity disorder (ADHD) on individuals and their families and provides insights into the neurobiological and environmental factors that contribute to ADHD while offering practical strategies for managing symptoms and improving well-being.

Tiny Habits: The Small Changes That Change Everything, by B. J. Fogg. This book offers a simple and accessible approach to developing new habits, with practical strategies for creating tiny habits that can lead to big changes.

Unwinding Anxiety: New Science Shows How to Break the Cycles of Worry and Fear to Heal Your Mind, by Judson Brewer. This book explores the science of anxiety and provides a mindfulness-based approach to managing it. The book offers practical strategies for identifying triggers and patterns of anxiety, and teaches readers how to use mindfulness to break the cycle of anxiety and develop healthier habits.

The Upward Spiral: Using Neuroscience to Reverse the Course of Depression, One Small Change at a Time, by Alex Korb. This book offers insights into the neuroscience of depression and provides practical strategies for improving mental health and well-being.

Waking the Tiger: Healing Trauma, by Peter A. Levine. This book provides insights into the neurobiology of trauma and offers practical strategies for healing trauma through somatic experiencing.

What Happened to You?: Conversations on Trauma, Resilience, and Healing, by Bruce D. Perry and Oprah Winfrey. This book helps you shift from asking the question "What's wrong with me?" to "What happened to me?" It discusses how our earliest experiences shape our lives, the impacts of trauma on the brain, and the many behavioral patterns we often struggle to understand.

When the Body Says No: Understanding the Stress-Disease Connection, by Gabor Maté. This book explores the link between stress and disease, with insights into how chronic stress can impact the nervous system and contribute to illness.

Why Has Nobody Told Me This Before?, by Julie Smith. This book is a practical guide to understanding your mental health struggles and provides a toolbox of skills to better navigate life's challenges and take charge of your mental health.

Why Zebras Don't Get Ulcers: An Updated Guide to Stress, Stress-Related Diseases, and Coping, by Robert M. Sapolsky. This book provides a comprehensive overview of the physiological effects of stress on the body and the nervous system and offers practical strategies for coping with stress.

Wearable Recommendations

Oura Ring: The Oura Ring tracks sleep, recovery, and activity. It measures physiological signals like heart rate, heart rate variability, and body temperature to provide overall health and well-being insights that are presented as a "score" alongside feedback on how to make improvements. This is the device I've been using for a couple of years now and love. Because it's a ring and not a wrist wearable, I find it much more comfortable to sleep with and wear 24/7, which gives me the most accurate overall data.

The following are wearable wrist devices with varying features, but all include tracking things mentioned in this book, including heart rate variability, physical activity, and sleep quality.

- WHOOP
- Apple Watch
- Fitbit
- Garmin

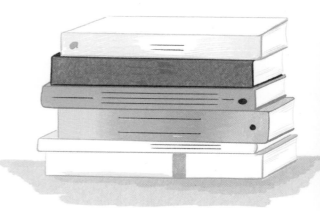

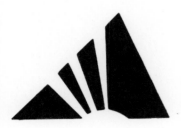

Rise As We Resources

Book Course

Visit www.riseaswe.com/vagusnerve for a guided video course that walks through this book with you and offers more resources, guided practices, and additional exercises to help you put what you're learning here into practice in your daily life.

Coaching Services

Visit www.riseaswe.com for more from Amanda and her team. Rise As We is a neuroscience-based, integrative, and trauma-informed coaching practice that helps individuals heal anxiety and depression through a lens of neuroscience, somatic parts work, and personalized lifestyle design. Head to their website to learn more about the variety of services offered and how you can receive personalized support on your own healing journey.

Podcast

Visit www.riseaswe.com/podcast, to tune in to Regulate & Rewire: An Anxiety and Depression Podcast, where we discuss the things I wish someone had taught me earlier in my healing journey. I share my steps, my missteps, and tangible, research-based tools to help you regulate your nervous system, rewire your mind, and reclaim your life.

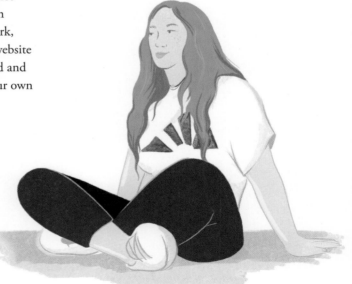

WORKS CITED

Amano, M., T. Kanda, H. Ue, and T. Moritani. "Exercise Training and Autonomic Nervous System Activity in Obese Individuals." *Medicine and Science in Sports and Exercise* 33, no. 8 (2001): 1287-91. doi:10.1097/00005768-200108000-00007

Bassi, Gabriel Shimizu, Daniel Penteado Martins Dias, Marcelo Franchin, Jhimmy Talbot, Daniel Gustavo Reis, Gustavo Batista Menezes, Jaci Airton Castania, Norberto Garcia-Cairasco, Leonardo Barbosa Moraes Resstel, Helo Cesar Slagado, et al. "Modulation of experimental arthritis by vagal sensory and central brain stimulation." *Brain, Behavior, and Immunity* 64 (April 2017): 330–343. doi:10.1016/j.bbi.2017.04.003

Beauchaine, Theodore. "Vagal Tone, Development, and Gray's Motivational Theory: Toward an Integrated Model of Autonomic Nervous System Functioning in Psychopathology." *Development and Psychopathology* 13, no. 2 (2001): 183–214. doi:10.1017/S0954579401002012

Ben-Menachem, E. (2001). "Vagus Nerve Stimulation, Side Effects, and Long-Term Safety." *Journal of Clinical Neurophysiology* 18 (September 2001): 415–418. doi: 10.1097/00004691-200109000-00005

Borges, Uirasso, Laura Knops, Sylvain Laborde, Stefanie Klatt, and Markus Raab. "Transcutaneous Vagus Nerve Stimulation May Enhance Only Specific Aspects of the Core Executive Functions: A Randomized Crossover Trial." *Frontiers in Neuroscience* 14 (May 2020): 1–18. doi: 10.3389/fnins.2020.00523

Borland, M.S., W.A. Vrana, N.A. Moreno, E.A. Fogarty, E.P. Buell, P. Sharma, C.T. Engineer, and M.P Kilgard. "Cortical Map Plasticity as a Function of Vagus Nerve Stimulation Intensity." *Brain Stimulation* 9, no. 1 (2016): 117–123. https://doi.org/10.1016/j.brs.2015.08.018

Borovikova, Lyudmila V., Svetlana Ivanova, Minghuang Zhang, Huan Yang, Galina I. Botchkina, Linda R. Watkins, Haichao Wang, Naji Abumrad, John W. Eaton, and Kevin J. Tracey. "Vagus Nerve Stimulation Attenuates the Systemic Inflammatory Response to Endotoxin." *Nature* 405 (2000): 458–462. https://doi.org/10.1038/35013070

Bush, Nicole R., Karen Jones-Mason, Michael Coccia, Zoe Caron, Abbey Alkon, Melanie Thomas, Kim Coleman-Phox, Pathik D. Wadhwa, Barbara A. Laraia, Nancy E. Adler, et al. "Effects of Pre- and Postnatal Maternal Stress on Infant Temperament and Autoimmune Nervous System Reactivity and Regulation in a Diverse, Low-Income Population." *Development and Psychopathology* 29, no. 5 (2017): 1553–1571. doi:10.1017/S0954579417001237

Cao, Bing, Jun Wang, Mahadi Shahed, Beth Jelfs, Rosa H. M. Chan, and Ying Li. "Vagus Nerve Stimulation Alters Phase Synchrony of the Anterior Cingulate Cortex and Facilitates Decision Making in Rats." *Scientific Reports* 6 (October 2016): 35135. https://doi.org/10.1038/srep35135

Carek, Peter J., Sarah E Laibstain, and Stephen M. Carek. "Exercise for the Treatment of Depression and Anxiety." *International Journal of Psychiatry in Medicine* 41, no. 1 (2011): 15–28. doi:10.2190/PM.41.1.c

Cechetto, David F. "Cortical Control of the Autonomic Nervous System." *Experimental Physiology* 99, no. 2 (2014): 326–331. doi:10.1113/expphysiol.2013.075192

Cerritelli, Francesco, Martin G. Frasch, Marta C. Antonelli, Chiara Viglione, Stefano Vecchi, Marco Chiera, and Andrea Manzotti. "A Review on the Vagus Nerve and Autonomic Nervous System During Fetal Development: Searching for Critical Windows." *Frontiers in Neuroscience* 15 (September 2021): 721605. doi:10.3389/fnins.2021.721605

Ceunen, Erik, Johan W. S. Vlaeyen, and Ilse Van Diest. "On the Origin of Interoception." *Frontiers in Psychology* 7 (May 2016): 743. doi:10.3389/fpsyg.2016.00743

Conway, Charles R., Arun Kumar, Willa Xiong, Mark Bunker, Scott T. Aaronson, and A. John Rush. "Chronic Vagus Nerve Stimulation Significantly Improves Quality of Life in Treatment-Resistant Major Depression." *The Journal of Clinical Psychiatry* 79, no. 5 (August 2018). doi:10.4088/JCP.18m12178

de Oliveira Ottone, Vinícius, Flávio de Castro Magalhães, Fabrício de Paula, Núbia Carelli Pereira Avelar, Paula Fernandes Aguiar, Pâmela Fiche da Matta Sampaio, Tamiris Campos Duarte, Karine Beatriz Costa, Tatiane Líliam Araújo, Cândido Celso Coimbra, et al. "The Effect of Different Water Immersion Temperatures on Post-Exercise Parasympathetic Reactivation." *PLOS One* 9, no. 12 (December 2014). doi:10.1371/journal.pone.0113730

Desbeaumes Jodoin, Véronique, François Richer, Jean-Phillipe Miron, Marie-Pierre Fournier-Gosselin, and Paul Lespérance. "Long-term Sustained Cognitive Benefits of Vagus Nerve Stimulation in Refractory Depression." *The Journal of ECT* 34, no. 4 (2018): 283–290. doi:10.1097/YCT.0000000000000502

Erman, Audrey B., Alexandra E. Kejner, Norman D. Hogikyan, and Eva L. Feldman. "Disorders of Cranial Nerves IX and X." *Seminars in Neurology* 29, no. 1 (2009): 85–92. doi:10.1055/s-0028-1124027

Gernot, Ernst. *Heart Rate Variability* (London: Springer-Verlag, 2014).

Haase, Lori, Jennifer L. Stewart, Brittany Youssef, April C. May, Sara Isakovic, Alan N. Simmons, Doughlas C. Johnson, Eric G. Potterat, and Martin P. Paulus. "When the Brain Does Not Adequately Feel the Body: Links Between Low Resilience and Interoception." *Biological Psychology* 113 (2016): 37–45. doi:10.1016/j.biopsycho.2015.11.004

Hayashi, N., Mutuhisa Ishihara, Ayumu Tanaka, Tomonori Osumi, and Takayoshi Yoshida. "Face Immersion Increases Vagal Activity as Assessed by Heart Rate Variability." *European Journal of Applied Physiology and Occupational Physiology* 76, no. 5 (1997): 394–399. doi:10.1007/s004210050267

Holochwost, Steven J., Jean-Louis Gariépy, Cathi B. Propper, W. Roger Mills-Koonce, and Ginger A. Moore. "Parenting Behaviors and Vagal Tone at Six Months Predict Attachment Disorganization at Twelve Months." *Developmental Psychobiology* 56, no. 6 (2014): 1423–1430. doi:10.1002/dev.21221

Kalyani, Bangalore G. Ganesan Venkatasubramanian, Rashmi Arasappa, Naren P. Rao, Sunil V. Kalmady, Rishikesh V. Behere, Hariprasad Rao, Mandapati K. Vasudev, and Bangalore N. Gangadhar. "Neurohemodynamic Correlates of 'OM' Chanting: A Pilot Functional Magnetic Resonance Imaging Study." *International Journal of Yoga* 4, no. 1 (2011): 3–6. doi:10.4103/0973-6131.78171

Kinoshita, Tomoko, Shinya Nagata, Reizo Baba, Takeshi Kohmoto, and Suketsune Iwagaki. "Cold-Water Face Immersion Per Se Elicits Cardiac Parasympathetic Activity." *Circulation Journal: Official Journal of the Japanese Circulation Society* 70, no. 6 (2006): 773–776. doi:10.1253/circj.70.773

Kulur, A. B., N. Haleagrahara, P. Adhikary, and P. S. Jeganathan. "Effect of Diaphragmatic Breathing on Heart Rate Variability in Ischemic Heart Disease with Diabetes." *Arquivos Brasileiros de Cardiologia* 92 no. 6 (June 2009): 423–499, 440–447, 457–463. doi: 10.1590/0066-782×2009000600008. PMID: 19629309

Liu, Longzhu, Ming Zhao, Xiaojiang Yu, and Weijin Zang. "Pharmacological Modulation of Vagal Nerve Activity in Cardiovascular Diseases." *Neuroscience Bulletin* 35, no. 1 (2019): 156–166. doi:10.1007/s12264-018-0286-7

Loper, Hailley, Monique Leinen, Logan Bassoff, Jack Sample, Mario Romero-Ortega, Kenneth J. Gustafson, Dawn M. Taylor, and Matthew A. Schiefer. "Both High Fat and High Carbohydrate Diets Impair Vagus Nerve Signaling of Satiety." *Scientific Reports* 11, no. 1 (May 2021): 10394. doi:10.1038/s41598-021-89465-0

McLaughlin, Katie A., Leslie Rith-Najarian, Melanie A. Dirks, and Margaret A. Sheridan. "Low Vagal Tone Magnifies the Association Between Psychosocial Stress Exposure and Internalizing Psychopathology in Adolescents." *Journal of Clinical Child & Adolescent Psychology* 44 no. 2 (October 2015): 314–328. doi:10.1080/15374416.2013.843464

Monk, Catherine, Richard P. Sloan, Michael M. Myers, Lauren Ellman, Elizabeth Werner, Jiyeon Jeon, Felice Tager, and William P. Fifer. "Fetal Heart Rate Reactivity Differs by Women's Psychiatric Status: An Early Marker for Developmental Risk?" *Journal of the American Academy of Child and Adolescent Psychiatry* 43, no. 3 (2004): 283–290. doi:10.1097/00004583-200403000-00009

Moore, Emma, Joel T. Fuller, Jonathan T. Buckley, Siena Saunders, Shona L. Halson, James R. Broatch, and Clint R. Bellenger. "Impact of Cold-Water Immersion Compared with Passive Recovery Following a Single Bout of Strenuous Exercise on Athletic Performance in Physically Active Participants: A Systematic Review with Meta-analysis and Meta-regression." *Sports Medicine (Auckland, N.Z.)* 52, no. 7 (2022): 1667–1688. doi:10.1007/s40279-022-01644-9

Moran, T. H., A. R. Baldessarini, C. F. Salorio, T. Lowery, and G. J. Schwartz. "Vagal Afferent and Efferent Contributions to the Inhibition of Food Intake by Cholecystokinin." *American Journal of Physiology* (1997). doi: 10.1152/ajpregu.1997.272.4.R1245

Nelson, Bryn. "Cannabis Conundrum: Evidence of Harm?: Opposition to Marijuana Use is Often Rooted in Arguments About the Drug's Harm to Children and Adults, but the Scientific Evidence is Seldom Clear-Cut." *Cancer Cytopathology* 123, no. 1 (2015): 1–2. doi:10.1002/cncy.21516

Neuhuber, Winfried L, and Hans-Rudolf Berthoud. "Functional Anatomy of the Vagus System: How Does the Polyvagal Theory Comply?" *Biological Psychology* 174 (2022): 108425. doi:10.1016/j.biopsycho.2022.108425

Paulus, Martin P., and Murray B. Stein. "Interoception in Anxiety and Depression." *Brain Structure & Function* 214, no. 5-6 (2010): 451–463. doi:10.1007/s00429-010-0258-9

Pellissier, Sonia, Cécile Dantzer, Laurie Mondillon, Candice Trocme, Anne-Sophie Gauchez, Véronique Ducros, Nicolas Mathiew, Bertrand Toussaint, Alicia Fornier, Frédéric Canini, et al. "Relationship Between Vagal Tone, Cortisol, TF-Alpha, Epinephrine and Negative Affects in Crohn's Disease and Irritable Bowel Syndrome." *PLOS One* 9, no. 9 (September 2014). doi:10.1371/journal.pone.0105328

Perini, Giulia Ida, Tommaso Toffanin, Giorgio Pigato, Giovanni Ferri, Halima Follador, Filippo Zonta, Carlo Pastorelli, Giulia Piazzon, Luca Denaro, Giussepe Rolma, et al. "Hippocampal Gray Volumes Increase in Treatment-Resistant Depression Responding to Vagus Nerve Stimulation." *The Journal of ECT* 33, no. 3 (2017): 160–166. doi:10.1097/YCT.0000000000000424

Porges, S. W. "Orienting in a Defensive World: Mammalian Modifications of Our Evolutionary Heritage: A Polyvagal Theory." *Psychophysiology* 32, no. 4 (1995): 301–318. doi:10.1111/j.1469-8986.1995.tb01213.x

Porges, Stephen W. "The Polyvagal Perspective." *Biological Psychology* 74, no. 2 (2007): 116–143. https://doi.org/10.1016/j.biopsycho.2006.06.009

Porges, Stephen W. "The Polyvagal Theory: New Insights into Adaptive Reactions of the Autonomic Nervous System." *Cleveland Clinic Journal of Medicine* 76, no. 2 (2009): doi:10.3949/ccjm.76.s2.17

Rash, Joshua A., Tavis S. Campbell, Nicole Letourneau, and Gerald F. Giesbrecht. "Maternal Cortisol during Pregnancy Is Related to Infant Cardiac Vagal Control." *Psychoneuroendocrinology* 54 (2015): 78–89. https://doi.org/10.1016/j.psyneuen.2015.01.024

Reed, Shawn F., Stephen W. Porges, and David B. Newlin. "Effect of Alcohol on Vagal Regulation of Cardiovascular Function: Contributions of the Polyvagal Theory to the Psychophysiology of Alcohol." *Experimental and Clinical Psychopharmacology* 7, no. 4 (1999): 484–492. doi:10.1037//1064-1297.7.4.484

Richer, Robert, Janis Zenkner, Arne Küderle, Nicolas Rohleder, and Bjoern M. Eskofier. "Vagus Activation by Cold Face Test Reduces Acute Psychosocial Stress Responses." *Scientific Reports* 12, no. 1 (November 2022). doi:10.1038/s41598-022-23222-9

Ritz, Thomas, Michelle Bosquet Enlow, Stefan M. Schulz, Robert Kitts, John Staudenmayer, and Rosalind J. Wright. "Respiratory Sinus Arrhythmia as an Index of Vagal Activity During Stress in Infants: Respiratory Influences and Their Control." *PLOS One* 7, no. 12 (2012). doi: 10.1371/journal.pone.0052729

Russo, Scott J., James W. Murrough, Ming-Hu Han, Dennis S. Charney, and Eric J. Nestler. "Neurobiology of Resilience." *Nature Neuroscience* 15, no. 11 (2012): 1475–1484. doi:10.1038/nn.3234

Sanders, Teresa H., Joseph Weiss, Luke Hogewood, Lan Chen, Casey Paton, Rebekah L. McMahan and J. David Sweatt. *Journal of Neuroscience* 39, no. 18 (May 2019): 3454–3469. doi:10.1523/jneurosci.2407-18.2019

Sandman, Curt A., Elysia P. Davis, Claudia Buss, and Laura M. Glynn. "Exposure to Prenatal Psychobiological Stress Exerts Programming Influences on the Mother and Her Fetus." *Neuroendocrinology* 95, no. 1 (2012): 7–21. doi:10.1159/000327017

Sandman, Curt A., Elysia P. Davis, Claudia Buss, and Laura M. Glynn. "Prenatal Programming of Human Neurological Function." *International Journal of Peptides* 2011 (2011). doi:10.1155/2011/837596

Sessa, Francesco, Valenzano Anna, Giovanni Messina, Giuseppe Cibelli, Vincenzo Monda, Gabriella Marsala, Maria Ruberto, Antonio Biondi, Orazio Cascio, Giuseppe Bertozzi, et al. "Heart Rate Variability as Predictive Factor for Sudden Cardiac Death." *Aging (Albany NY)* 10, no. 2 (February 2018): 166–177 doi:10.18632/aging./01386

Steffen, Patrick R., Derek Bartlett, Rachel Marie Channell, Katelyn Jackman, Mikel Cressman, John Bills, and Meredith Pescatello. "Integrating Breathing Techniques Into Psychotherapy to Improve HRV: Which Approach Is Best?" *Journal of Frontiers in Psychology* 12 (2021). doi:10.3389/ "Cognition-Enhancing Vagus Nerve Stimulation Alters the Epigenetic Landscape." fpsyg.2021.624254

Thayer, J. F., and R. D. Lane. "A Model of Neurovisceral Integration in Emotion Regulation and Dysregulation." *Journal of Affective Disorders* 61, no. 3 (2000): 201–216. doi:10.1016/s0165-0327(00)00338-4

Thayer, Julian F., and Richard D. Lane. "The Role of Vagal Function in the Risk for Cardiovascular Disease and Mortality." *Biological Psychology* 74, no. 2 (2007): 224–242. doi:10.1016/j.biopsycho.2005.11.013

Tindle, Jacob, and Prasanna Tadi. "Neuroanatomy, Parasympathetic Nervous System." *National Library of Medicine* (2022). https://www.ncbi.nlm.nih.gov/books/ NBK553141/

van de Wall E. H. E. M., P. Duffy, and R. C. Ritter. "CCK Enhances Response to Gastric Distension by Acting on Capsaicin-Insensitive Vagal Afferents." *American Journal of Physiology-Regulatory, Integrative and Comparative Physiology* 289, no. 3 (September 2005): 695–703. doi:10.1152/ ajpregu.00809.2004

Vidotto, Laís Silva, Celso Ricardo Fernandes de Carvalho, Alex Harvey, and Mandy Jones. "Dysfunctional Breathing: What Do We Know?" *The Brazilian Journal of Pulmonology* 45, no. 1 (February 2019). doi:10.1590/1806-3713/ e20170347

Waxenbaum, Joshua A., Vamsi Reddy, and Matthew Varacallo. "Anatomy, Autonomic Nervous System." StatPearls Publishing, Treasure Island, FL, January 2023. https://www. ncbi.nlm.nih.gov/books/NBK539845/

Zaccaro, Andrea, Andrea Piarulli, Marco Laurino, Erika Garbella, Danilo Menicucci, Bruno Neri, and Angelo Gemignani. "How Breath-Control Can Change Your Life: A Systematic Review on Psycho-Physiological Correlates of Slow Breathing." *Frontiers in Human Neuroscience* 12 (September 2018): 353. doi:10.3389/fnhum.2018.00353

Zhang, Han, Zhiwei Guo, Yun Qu, Yu Zhao, Yuxuan Yang, Juan De, and Chunlan Yang. "Cognitive Function and Brain Activation Before and After Transcutaneous Cervical Vagus Nerve Stimulation in Healthy Adults: A Concurrent tcVNS-fMRI Study." *Frontiers in Psychology* 13 (2022). doi:10.3389/ fpsyg.2022.1003411

Zulfiqar, Usman, Donald A. Jurivich, Weihua Gao, and Donald H. Singer. "Relation of High Heart Rate Variability to Healthy Longevity." *The American Journal of Cardiology* 105, no. 8 (2010): 1181–1185. doi:10.1016/j. amjcard.2009.12.022

ABOUT THE AUTHOR

AMANDA ARMSTRONG is the founder and CEO of Rise As We, an integrative mental health practice with a specialty in helping clients struggling with anxiety and depression. Amanda's unique approach combines her certified professional and trauma-informed coach training with a master's degree in kinesiology (exercise psychology) and a previous career in the corporate wellness space at Google HQ. She draws on all this experience to help her clients heal through a nervous system–based approach that gives mental and physical health an equal seat at the table.

In addition to her private practice, Amanda is a wife, mother, podcast host, and speaker who hosts workshops and lectures on nervous system–based mental health support. You can connect with her and learn more at riseaswe.com.

ACKNOWLEDGMENTS

To my editor, Thom; the incredible team at Quarto; and my illustrator, Eleanor: Thank you for bringing this book to life in such an impactful and beautiful way.

To my Rise As We team, family, friends, and fellow practitioners who cheered me on and supported me every step of the way. Writing a book with my pregnancy proving a strict deadline was no easy feat. And to my clients: I've learned so much from and with each of you, and that helped shape this book. It's an absolute honor to be invited into your healing journey.

To my husband, Christopher, and our three sons—the one earthside, the one we lost, and the one on the way—you are the loves of my life and my deepest inspiration. You have been the catalyst for so much of my own healing and are my most dedicated and enthusiastic fans. Thanks for your unwavering support, the reminders of just how capable I am, and a shared enthusiasm for how important the work I do is in the world.

INDEX